Handbook of Skin Disease Management

Handbook of Skin Disease Management

Zainab Jiyad
Consultant Dermatologist
St George's Hospital
London, UK

Honorary Senior Lecturer
Population Health Research Institute
St George's University of London
London, UK

Carsten Flohr
Honorary Consultant Dermatologist
Guys and St Thomas' NHS Foundation Trust
London, UK

Chair in Dermatology and Population Health Sciences
St John's Institute of Dermatology
King's College London
London, UK

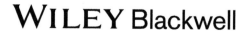

Registered Offices
John Wiley & Sons, Inc., 111 River Street, Hoboken, NJ 07030, USA
John Wiley & Sons Ltd, The Atrium, Southern Gate, Chichester, West Sussex, PO19 8SQ, UK

For details of our global editorial offices, customer services, and more information about Wiley products visit us at www.wiley.com.

Library of Congress Cataloging-in-Publication Data Applied for

Paperback: 9781119829041

Cover Design: Wiley
Cover Images: © Vandathai/Shutterstock

Set in 9.5/12.5pt STIXTwoText by Straive, Pondicherry, India
Printed and bound by CPI Group (UK) Ltd, Croydon, CR0 4YY

C9781119829041_040123

Contents

Expert Contributors

We would like to thank the following contributors for their expertise in reviewing and modifying the content.

Wedad Abdelrahman
Bullous pemphigoid, dermatitis herpetiformis, linear IgA disease, and pemphigus vulgaris and foliaceus
St John's Institute of Dermatology, Guy's and St Thomas' NHS Foundation Trust, London

Alya Abdul-Wahab
Hyperhidrosis and pigmented purpuric dermatosis
St George's University Hospitals NHS Foundation Trust, London

Victoria Akhras
Dermatomyositis, lupus erythematosus, melanoma, polyarteritis nodosa, and vasculitis
St George's University Hospitals NHS Foundation Trust, London

Emma Amoafo
Hair in skin of colour (appendix)
St George's University Hospitals NHS Foundation Trust, London

Nelomi Anandagoda
Pruritus and calciphylaxis
Guy's and St Thomas' NHS Foundation Trust, London

Jonathan Batchelor
Vitiligo
King's College Hospital NHS Foundation Trust, London

Anthony Bewley
Psychodermatology
Queen Mary University of London and Barts Health NHS Trust, London

Tanya Bleiker
Grover's disease
University Hospitals of Derby and Burton, Derby

Siobhan Carey
Content, overall review, and appendix
St John's Institute of Dermatology, Guy's and St Thomas' NHS Foundation Trust, London

Carmen Chang
Lipodermatosclerosis, lymphoedema,
and leg ulcers
*St George's University Hospitals NHS
Foundation Trust, London*

David De Berker
Lichen planus
*University Hospitals Bristol and
Weston NHS Foundation Trust,
Bristol*

Leila Ferguson
Granuloma annulare and molluscum
contagiosum
*St George's University Hospitals
NHS Foundation Trust,
London*

Charlotte Fleming
Chilblains and papular urticaria
*St George's University Hospitals NHS
Foundation Trust, London*

Patryk Gawrysiak
Lipodermatosclerosis, lymphoedema,
and leg ulcers
*St George's University Hospitals NHS
Foundation Trust, London*

Kristiana Gordon
Lipodermatosclerosis, lymphoedema,
and leg ulcers
*St George's University Hospitals NHS
Foundation Trust, London*

Clive Grattan
Mastocytosis, urticaria, and urticarial
vasculitis
*St John's Institute of Dermatology,
Guy's and St Thomas' NHS Foundation
Trust, London*

Christopher Griffiths
Psoriasis
University of Manchester, Manchester

Matthew Harries
Alopecia areata, folliculitis decalvans,
and lichen planopilaris
*Northern Care Alliance NHS
Foundation Trust, Salford*

Catherine Harwood
Actinic keratosis, erosive pustular
dermatosis, and porokeratosis
*Queen Mary University of London and
Barts Health NHS Trust, London*

Roderick Hay
Scabies
King's College London, London

Bernard Ho
Lipodermatosclerosis, lymphoedema,
and leg ulcers
*St George's University Hospitals NHS
Foundation Trust, London*

Anthony Hulse
Acanthosis nigricans and hirsutism
*Evelina London Children's Hospital,
Guy's and St Thomas' NHS Foundation
Trust, London*

Sally Ibbotson
Chronic actinic dermatitis and
polymorphic light eruption
University of Dundee, Dundee

Arvind Kaul
Dermatomyositis and lupus
erythematosus
*St George's University Hospitals NHS
Foundation Trust, London*

Samantha Keegan
Bowen's disease, SCC
*St George's University Hospitals NHS
Foundation Trust, London*

Imran Khan
Essential lists (appendix)
*St George's University Hospitals NHS
Foundation Trust, London*

Ruth Lamb
Hidradenitis suppurative and
systemics/biologics
*St George's University Hospitals NHS
Foundation Trust, London*

Alison Layton
Acne
*Skin Research Centre, University of
York, York*

Laurence Le Cleach
Lichen planus
Henri Mondor Hospital, Créteil

Haur Yueh Lee
Drug reactions and erythema
multiforme
*Singapore General Hospital,
Singapore*

Fiona Lewis
Lichen sclerosus
*St John's Institute of Dermatology,
Guy's and St Thomas' NHS Foundation
Trust, London*

Sue Lewis-Jones
Pityriasis lichenoides
*Ninewells Hospital, Dundee
(Retired)*

Jemima Mellerio
Darier disease, pityriasis rubra pilaris,
and zinc deficiency
*St John's Institute of Dermatology,
Guy's and St Thomas' NHS Foundation
Trust, London*

Rachael Morris-Jones
Fungal skin infections, folliculitis,
pityriasis versicolor, and
pseudofolliculitis barbae
*St John's Institute of Dermatology,
Guy's and St Thomas' NHS Foundation
Trust, London*

Celia Moss
Ichthyosis and keratosis pilaris
*Birmingham Women's and Children's
NHS Foundation Trust, Birmingham*

Ruth Murphy
Behcet's
*Sheffield Teaching Hospitals NHS
Foundation Trust and Sheffield
University, Sheffield*

Eugene Ong
Pruritus and sarcoidosis
*St George's University Hospitals NHS
Foundation Trust, London*

Tony Ormerod
Pyoderma gangrenosum
University of Aberdeen, Aberdeen

Catherine Orteu
Morphea
*Centre for Rheumatology and
Connective Tissue Diseases, Royal
Free London NHS Foundation
Trust, London*

Lucy Ostlere
Contact dermatitis
St George's University Hospitals NHS Foundation Trust, London

Edel O'Toole
Palmoplantar keratoderma
Queen Mary University of London and Barts Health NHS Trust, London

Rakesh Patalay
Keloid, lentigo maligna, and melasma
St John's Institute of Dermatology, Guy's and St Thomas' NHS Foundation Trust, London

Mark Pearson
Lipodermatosclerosis, lymphoedema, and leg ulcers
St George's University Hospitals NHS Foundation Trust, London

Vanessa Pinder
Hailey-Hailey
Epsom and St Helier University Hospitals NHS Trust, London

Venura Samarasinghe
BCC and chondrodermatitis nodularis helicis chronicus
St George's University Hospitals NHS Foundation Trust, London

Jane Setterfield
Aphthous ulcers
St John's Institute of Dermatology, Guy's and St Thomas' NHS Foundation Trust, London

Julia Soo
Vulvodynia
Epsom and St Helier University Hospitals NHS Trust and St George's University Hospitals NHS Foundation Trust, London

Catherine M. Stefanato
Alopecia biopsy (appendix)
St John's Institute of Dermatology, Guy's and St Thomas' NHS Foundation Trust, London

Jane Sterling
Warts
Cambridge University Hospitals NHS Foundation Trust, Cambridge

Yishi Tan
Graft-versus-host disease
Guy's and St Thomas' NHS Foundation Trust, London

Christos Tziotzios
Central centrifugal cicatricial alopecia, dissecting cellulitis of the scalp, and male pattern hair loss
St John's Institute of Dermatology, Guy's and St Thomas' NHS Foundation Trust, London

Esther van Zuuren
Rosacea
Leiden University Medical Center, Leiden

Mary Wain
Mycosis fungoides
St John's Institute of Dermatology, Guy's and St Thomas' NHS Foundation Trust, London

Dmitri Wall
Acne keloidalis, female pattern hair loss, and telogen effluvium
University College Dublin, Hair Restoration Blackrock, and the Mater Misericordiae University Hospital, Dublin

Jamie Wee
Erythema nodosum and Sweet's syndrome
Ng Teng Fong General Hospital, Singapore

Preface

At some stage in dermatology, one will find that the difficulty of managing conditions can overtake the diagnostic challenge. Whilst a plethora of studies, review articles, and expert opinions are published on a daily basis, staying up-to-date with these and applying them in a practical manner is incredibly difficult.

As such, it was our intention to create a handbook with emphasis on best evidence, making as much use of clinical guidelines and systematic reviews/meta-analyses as possible, whilst remaining close to 'real-world' clinical practice.

Each condition is presented as succinctly as possible, occupying no more than a couple of pages. This book is intended to be used 'on the move', in clinic, on the wards, and in the lecture theatre, with dermatology trainees and consultants in mind, as well as GPs.

We are grateful to our expert reviewers and contributors for their recommendations, suggestions, and expertise.

We hope that this book will serve as a succinct management guide for those dealing with skin disease.

ZJ and CF

Abbreviations

5-FU	5 Fluorouracil
5-HIAA	5-hydroxyindoleacetic acid
A&E	Accident and emergency
AA	Alopecia areata
ABPI	Ankle brachial pressure index
ACE	Angiotensin converting enzyme
AD	Atopic dermatitis
AGEP	Acute generalised exanthematous pustulosis
AJCC	American joint committee on cancer
AK	Actinic keratosis
ALT	Alanine transaminase
ANA	Antinuclear antibodies
ANCA	Antineutrophil cytoplasmic antibodies
ARCI	Autosomal recessive congenital ichthyosis
ASOT	Anti-streptolysin O titre
AST	Aspartate transaminase
AZA	Azathioprine
BCC	Basal cell carcinoma
BD	Twice daily
BP	Blood pressure
Bx	Biopsy
C&C	Curettage and cautery
CAD	Chronic actinic dermatitis
CADM	Clinically amyopathic dermatomyositis
CAH	Congenital adrenal hyperplasia
CBT	Cognitive behaviour therapy
CCCA	Central centrifugal cicatricial alopecia

CDASI	Cutaneous dermatomyositis disease area and severity index
CDLQI	Children's dermatology life quality index
CK	Creatine kinase
CLASI	Cutaneous lupus erythematosus disease area and severity index
CMV	Cytomegalovirus
CNS	Central nervous system
COCP	Combined oral contraceptive pill
CRP	C-reactive protein
CS	Corticosteroid
CsA	Ciclosporin
CSU	Chronic spontaneous urticaria
CTCL	Cutaneous T cell lymphoma
CTD	Connective tissue disease
CXR	Chest x-ray
DH	Dermatitis herpetiformis
DHEAS	Dehydroepiandrosterone sulfate
DLCO	Diffusing capacity for carbon monoxide
DLI	Donor lymphocyte infusions
DLQI	Dermatology life quality index
DM	Dermatomyositis
DPCP	Diphenylcyclopropenone
DRESS	Drug reaction with eosinophilia and systemic symptoms
EASI	Eczema area and severity index
EB	Epidermolysis bullosa
EBV	Epstein-Barr virus
ECG	Electrocardiogram
ECP	Extracorporeal photophoresis
EGFR	Estimated glomerular filtration rate
EM	Erythema multiforme
EMG	Electromyography
EN	Erythema nodosum
ENA	Extractable nuclear antigen
EPD	Erosive pustular dermatosis
EPDS	Erosive pustular dermatosis of the scalp
ESR	Erythrocyte sedimentation rate
F-G	Ferriman-Gallwey
FBC	Full blood count

FFA	Frontal fibrosing alopecia
FNA	Fine needle aspiration
FSH	Follicle-stimulating hormone
FT	Field treatment
G6PD	Glucose-6-phosphate dehydrogenase
GFD	Gluten free diet
GFR	Glomerular filtration rate
GI	Gastrointestinal
GTN	Glyceryl trinitrate
GVHD	Graft-versus-host disease
Hb	Haemoglobin
HHV	Human herpesvirus
HiSCR	Hidradenitis suppurativa clinical response
HIV	Human immunodeficiency virus
HRCT	High-resolution computerised tomography
HRT	Hormone replacement therapy
HS	Hidradenitis suppurativa
HSV	Herpes simplex virus
HUVS	Hypocomplementaemic urticarial vasculitis syndrome
Hx	History
IBD	Inflammatory bowel disease
ICBD	International criteria for Behçet's disease
IH	Infantile haemangioma
IL	Intralesional
ILD	Interstitial lung disease
IMF	Immunofluorescence
IPL	Intense pulsed light
ISG	International study group
IUD	Intrauterine device
IVIG	Intravenous immunoglobulin
JAK	Janus kinase
KOH	Potassium hydroxide
KP	Keratosis pilaris
KTP	Potassium titanyl phosphate
LDH	Lactate dehydrogenase
LDOM	Low-dose oral minoxidil
LDS	Lipodermatosclerosis

LDT	Lesion directed treatment
LE	Lupus erythematosus
LFTs	Liver function tests
LH	Luteinising hormone
LLLT	Low-level laser light therapy
LM	Lentigo maligna
LP	Lichen planus
LPP	Lichen planopilaris
LS	Lichen sclerosus
MA	Meta-analysis
MAA	Myositis-associated antibody
MASI	Melasma area and severity index
MCV	Mean corpuscular volume
MDS	Myelodysplastic syndrome
MDT	Multidisciplinary team
MGUS	Monoclonal gammopathy of undetermined significance
MLD	Manual lymphatic drainage
MMF	Mycophenolate mofetil
MMS	Mohs micrographic surgery
MPCM	Maculopapular cutaneous mastocytosis
MRI	Magnetic resonance imaging
MSA	Myositis-specific antibody
mSWAT	Modified severity-weighted assessment tool
MTX	Methotrexate
NAPSI	Nail psoriasis severity index
NBUVB	Narrowband UVB
NCCN	National comprehensive cancer network
NICE	National institute for health and care excellence
NOACs	Novel oral anticoagulants
NSAID	Non-steroidal anti-inflammatory drugs
OCP	Oral contraceptive pill
OD	Once daily
OT	Occupational therapy
PAN	Polyarteritis nodosa
PASI	Psoriasis area severity index
PCOS	Polycystic ovary syndrome
PDT	Photodynamic therapy

PEST	Psoriasis epidemiology screening tool
PFT	Pulmonary function test
PG	Pyoderma gangrenosum
PGA	Physician global assessment
PLE	Polymorphic light eruption
POEM	Patient oriented eczema measure
PRP	Pityriasis rubra pilaris
PsA	Psoriatic arthritis
PTH	Parathyroid hormone
PUVA	Psoralen ultraviolet A
RA	Rheumatoid arthritis
RCT	Randomised controlled trial
RR	Relative risk
SADBE	Squaric acid dibutyl ester
SC	Subcutaneous
SCAR	Severe cutaneous adverse reactions
SCC	Squamous cell carcinoma
SCLE	Subcutaneous lupus erythematosus
SCORAD	SCORing Atopic Dermatitis
SHBG	Sex hormone binding globulin
SJS	Stevens-Johnson syndrome
SLE	Systemic lupus erythematosus
SNB	Sentinel node biopsy
SR	Systematic review
SSRI	Selective serotonin reuptake inhibitors
STS	Sodium thiosulphate
TB	Tuberculosis
TCS	Topical corticosteroid
TDS	Three times a day
TEN	Toxic epidermal necrolysis
TFTs	Thyroid function tests
TMEP	Telangiectasia macularis eruptiva perstans
TNF	Tumour necrosis factor
TNM	Tumour nodes metastasis
TPMT	Thiopurine methyltransferase
Tx	Treatment
U/Es	Urea and electrolytes

UC	Ulcerative colitis
UP	Urticaria pigmentosa
URTI	Upper respiratory tract infection
US	Ultrasound
UV	Urticarial vasculitis
VIP	Vasoactive intestinal peptide
VZV	Varicella zoster virus
WBC	White blood cell
WLE	Wide local excision

How to Use This Book

Treatments are listed in numerical steps. A key concept of skin disease management is combining or 'stacking' treatments. As such, we have opted for the terms 'steps' as opposed to 'first-line, second-line' to reflect the concept of treatments building on each other.

Next to each treatment you will see a number (1–4). This is the grade for each treatment modality, according to the best available evidence, adapted from the Oxford Levels of Evidence, below. It clearly makes a big difference when prescribing treatment based on case reports, as opposed to a meta-analysis of several robust randomised controlled trials. We feel it is vital that both clinicians and patients understand where the advice for treatment comes from.

1	Best evidence from meta-analysis of randomised controlled trials
2	Best evidence from randomised controlled trial(s)
3	Best evidence from uncontrolled study/studies
4	Best evidence from case report/series or expert opinion

The appendix section at the end covers most clinic essentials – initiation and monitoring of systemics as well how to manage abnormal results, essential lists (e.g. causes of panniculitis), topical treatments, hepatitis B serology, alopecia in skin of colour management tips, and more.

About the Companion Website

This book is accompanied by a companion website:

www.wiley.com/go/jiyad/handbookofskindiseasemanagement

The website includes:

- References

Acanthosis nigricans

The vast majority of cases are due to insulin-resistant states, where the condition is often termed 'pseudoacanthosis nigricans', contrasting with cases of 'true' acanthosis nigricans due to an underlying malignancy.

All Patients

1) **Take history screening for underlying causes:** obesity, diabetes, PCOS, malignancy (usually GI or ovarian), familial, drugs (e.g. steroids), and any other causes of insulin resistance.
2) **Perform focused examination screening for above.**
3) **Investigations:** blood pressure, lipid profile, HBA1C; other investigations as per hx.
4) **Encourage weight loss:** there is evidence to show this can improve acanthosis nigricans.

Red-flags that suggest underlying malignancy: rapid onset, old age at onset, absence of obesity or cause of insulin resistance, unintentional weight loss, tripe palms, extensive involvement.

Step 1

- **Topical retinoids alone or in triple cream combinations** [4]: *most commonly used.* In an RCT comparing tretinoin with adapalene, at least 85% of participants in both groups had >75% improvement on investigator's global evaluation. Use OD, as tolerated. Triple combination creams with topical steroid and hydroxychloroquine have been used with success in case reports (e.g. Pigmanorm®).
- **Topical vitamin D analogues** [4]: use calcipotriol BD.
- **Keratolytics** [4]: in an RCT comparing 10% urea vs tretinoin, both showed improvement, although tretinoin performed significantly better.

Handbook of Skin Disease Management, First Edition. Zainab Jiyad and Carsten Flohr.
© 2023 John Wiley & Sons Ltd. Published 2023 by John Wiley & Sons Ltd.
Companion website: www.wiley.com/go/jiyad/handbookofskindiseasemanagement

Step 2

- **Oral retinoids** [4]: isotretinoin and acitretin (<u>variable doses</u>) have both been used in case reports, but relapse on stopping treatment has occurred.
- **Metformin** [4]: RCT (n=33) of metformin vs alpha-lipoic acid, showed significant improvement in both groups.
- **Laser treatments** [4]: erbium, alexandrite, and CO_2 lasers have all been used with success.

Refractory

- **Chemical peels** [3]: in 6 women, 15% TCA peels applied <u>once/week for 4 weeks</u> showed improvement in all.
- **Others:** octreotide, PUVA.

Acne keloidalis nuchae

Some believe that early aggressive treatment with surgery is a preferable strategy to prevent progression, but most would follow a traditional approach beginning with topical therapy.

Encourage all patients to avoid exacerbating factors

- Hats/helmets/bands over the site.
- Shaving and tight hair grooming practices.

Step 1

Often the following treatments are combined:

- **Potent/superpotent TCS/IL steroids** [3]: some begin with topical applications <u>OD</u>, whilst many initiate with IL steroids <u>(10–40mg/mL) approximately every 6 weeks.</u>
- **Topical antibiotics** [4]: topical clindamycin commonly used <u>OD.</u>
- **Topical retinoids** [4]: can cause irritation so best used in conjunction with steroids. Use <u>OD.</u>

Step 2

- **Tetracyclines** [4]: <u>lymecycline 408mg OD or doxycycline 100mg OD/BD</u> widely used. Evidence from case reports and expert opinion.

Step 3

- **Lasers** [3]: a pilot study of 16 patients treated with 5 sessions of long-pulsed Nd:YAG laser reported an 82% mean improvement. Various other laser methods have been utilitised with success including alexandrite and 810-nm diode.
- **Isotretinoin** [4]: case reports to suggest treatment success. It is likely that low doses are all that is required, <u>consider initiating and maintaining at 20mg OD.</u>

Refractory

- **Surgery** [3]: in a study of 25 who underwent surgical excision, all reported good–excellent cosmetic outcome but 15 developed papules and pustules within the scar. Deep punch biopsies and secondary-intention healing has been used for removal of papules. CO_2 laser has been used for laser excision.
- **Others:** cryotherapy, UV light, and radiotherapy.

Handbook of Skin Disease Management, First Edition. Zainab Jiyad and Carsten Flohr.
© 2023 John Wiley & Sons Ltd. Published 2023 by John Wiley & Sons Ltd.
Companion website: www.wiley.com/go/jiyad/handbookofskindiseasemanagement

Acne vulgaris

Disease severity is multifactorial and dictates the initiating step for treatment selection. Severe acne is defined clinically as acne conglobata, nodulocystic acne, or acne at risk of permanent scarring that has not responded to combination therapy that includes an antimicrobial treatment. Scarring acne should be treated aggressively to avoid permanent physical and psychological sequelae. Comorbidities including endocrinopathies should be factored into treatment decisions, as should the impact of acne on mental health.

All Patients

1) Assess **psychosocial impact**, refer to mental health specialists as appropriate.
2) Consider **the extent and duration** of acne as well as the response to previous treatment.
3) Assess for **scarring and pigmentation** to allow for early effective therapy to mitigate these sequelae.
4) Note the degree of **seborrhoea** as high sebum correlates with a poor response to antibiotics.
5) Explain **treatment options** and signpost to appropriate patient information and support, e.g. acnesupport.org.uk.
6) Provide **clear instructions** on how to use therapies and encourage good adherence.
7) Recommend **gentle cleansing** and **avoidance of comedogenic** products as a means of supporting treatment tolerability.
8) Consider underlying **comorbidities**, e.g. endocrinopathies associated with androgen excess or drug-induced disease.

Handbook of Skin Disease Management, First Edition. Zainab Jiyad and Carsten Flohr.
© 2023 John Wiley & Sons Ltd. Published 2023 by John Wiley & Sons Ltd.
Companion website: www.wiley.com/go/jiyad/handbookofskindiseasemanagement

> ### Step 1

Combination topicals outperform single agents consistently in RCTs ①: principals of treatment include use of combination topical retinoid and antimicrobial treatments, and avoidance of antibiotics as monotherapy.

- **Any severity:** fixed combination topical adapalene with benzoyl peroxide (Epiduo®), or tretinoin with clindamycin (Treclin®), *use daily – alternate day and short contact use may support tolerability as would the use of good skin care regimens.*
- **Mild to moderate combination benzoyl peroxide with topical clindamycin** (Duac Once Daily®).
- **Topical benzoyl peroxide monotherapy** could be used as an alternative treatment to the fixed combinations if these treatments are contraindicated, or the patient wishes to avoid using a topical retinoid or an antibiotic (topical or oral).

> ### Step 2

For moderate to severe disease, topical nonantibiotic agents plus systemic antibiotics can be considered:

- **Oral tetracycline with non-antibiotic topicals** ①: fixed combination topical adapalene and benzoyl peroxide (Epiduo®) plus an oral tetracycline lymecycline 408mg OD or doxycycline 100mg OD. Minocycline is widely used in US, but potential severe side effects and cost have limited UK availability. Azelaic acid (Skinoren®, Finacea®) is an alternative second-line topical applied twice daily and used in combination with an oral tetracycline.
- **Alternative (second-line) antibiotic with non-antibiotic topical** ②: (if tetracyclines contraindicated) plus a non-antibiotic topical. Macrolides, e.g. erythromycin (500mg BD 12 weeks). Less commonly, trimethoprim (caution severe cutaneous adverse drug reactions) 200–300mg BD 12 weeks.
- **Combined oral contraceptive pill (COCP)** ①: no single COCP has performed better and a Cochrane review found all worked for treating inflammatory acne. A meta-analysis has shown similar efficacy to oral antibiotics at 6 months. Consider COCP risk and combine with isotretinoin/tetracycline for contraceptive use.

> ### Refractory

- **Isotretinoin** ①: *see page 189 for dose, initiation, and managing complications.* In severe cystic acne, oral ***prednisolone,*** *e.g. 20mg as reducing dose over 4 weeks, can be considered to* prevent severe initial flare.
- **Spironolactone** ①: there is currently no robust evidence for spironolactone to treat acne in adult females. However, there are case series and some retrospective studies suggesting benefit in this population. A large NIHR HTA prospective study has been recently conducted examining the use of oral spironolactone in adult female acne; results are awaited. *See page 193 for dosing.*

Acne relapses after isotretinoin

- **Consider those patients likely to relapse,** e.g. younger patients, those with truncal acne, family history of severe acne, those with potential endocrinopathies or androgen excess – consider investigating for the latter.
- **Consider maintenance therapy with combination topical retinoid and benzoyl peroxide,** in those patients at high risk of relapse.

Clinical pearls

- **Alternate-day topical retinoid application and short contact use** can mitigate adverse effects.
- **Good skin care regimens support adherence.**
- **Antibiotics topical and oral should not be used as monotherapy.**
- **Judicious use of antibiotics** will reduce the likelihood of antimicrobial resistance.
- **Gram negative folliculitis** can occur due to long-term antibiotic use. Consider this in patients who develop multiple pustules after a good response or who develop a deterioration of their acne. Assess swabs for microbiology. The treatment of choice for this is isotretinoin.
- **Low-dose isotretinoin at start of treatment** is associated with less acne flare.
- **Isotretinoin is better absorbed with food:** ensure patients take it with food, ideally fatty food, to improve efficacy. Taking isotretinoin on empty stomach can reduce absorption by up to 60%.
- **Triamcinolone injections:** can be very useful for severe acne nodules/cysts.

Managing scarring/post-inflammatory pigmentation

- **Different treatments reported for different scar types:** see table below.
- **Hyperpigmentation tx options:** sun protection, topical retinoid, azelaic acid, topical hydroquinone (combination creams like Pigmanorm® can be trialled), chemical peels.

Efficacy of modalities per atrophic scar type

Type of treatment	Modality[a]	Icepick scars	Rolling scars	Shallow boxcar scars	Deep boxcar scars
Resurfacing	Microdermabrasion				
	Dermabrasion				
	Peels				
	CROSS				
	Needling				
	Ablative laser				
Lifting-related	Subcision				
Volume-related	Filler				
	Platelet-rich plasma[b]				
Skin tightening	Fractional/nonablative lasers				
	Fractional radiofrequency				
Surgery/movement-related	Punch elevation				
	Punch excision				

Effective　　Less effective　　Ineffective

CROSS chemical reconstruction of skin scars.
[a]Modalities with substantial quality of evidence data are included.
[b]Used as adjunct to other procedures.

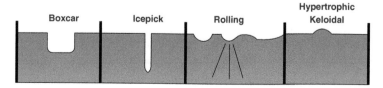

Boxcar　　Icepick　　Rolling　　Hypertrophic Keloidal

Source: Bhargava S, Cunha PR, Lee J, Kroumpouzos G. Acne scarring management: systematic review and evaluation of the evidence. Am J Clin Dermatol 2018;19(4):459–77.

Actinic keratosis (AK)

Although the majority of cutaneous SCCs (cSCCs) arise from AKs, the risk of malignant transformation of an individual AK is uncertain and reported as 0.075–0.1%. It is not always appropriate or feasible to treat all AKs. But treatment vs no treatment and the type of treatment used should be considered on a case-by-case basis with the patient. Sun protection is routinely advised.

- **Lesion directed treatment (LDT) vs field treatment (FT):** AKs that are confluent in an area >1cm^2 with subclinical dysplasia (field change) are at high risk for progression to cSCC and FT is preferrable to LDT alone, although both may be used together.

- **5-Fluorouracil (5-FU) cream** ③: FT (and LDT). *Use first-line.* In a multicentre RCT of 624 participants, 5-FU was more effective than imiquimod, ingenol mebutate, and MAL-PDT. Variable regimens used: OD/BD for 2–4 weeks as standard but alternatives include, e.g. 3 times a week for 8–12 weeks. Often used with TCS–antibiotic combination to reduce local skin reactions (redness, crusting, discomfort). Available in combination with salicylic acid for LDT of hypertrophic AK. Shorter treatment courses (4 days) also described when used in combination with calcipotriol ointment.
- **Cryotherapy** ③: LDT. Rapid tx makes this a popular option. A SR reported a response rate varying from 39 to 76%. Warn of the risk of blistering, scarring, and pigment change.
- **Imiquimod cream** ③: FT. Applied 3 times a week at night for 4 weeks. Local skin reactions usually occur.
- **Surgery** ④: LDT. Generally reserved for hypertrophic AKs, where other treatments have failed, or to confirm the diagnosis and exclude cSCC. Usually curettage and cautery or shave excision.
- **Ingenol mebutate gel** ①: FT. *Used OD for 2–3 days. At the time of publication, prescribing is suspended in Europe and Canada due to the possible increased risk of cSCC, which is undergoing investigation.*
- **Diclofenac/hyaluronic acid gel:** FT. Used BD for 60–90 days with milder local skin reactions than 5-FU and imiquimod but generally reduced efficacy, although few head-to-head clinical trials.

Handbook of Skin Disease Management, First Edition. Zainab Jiyad and Carsten Flohr.
© 2023 John Wiley & Sons Ltd. Published 2023 by John Wiley & Sons Ltd.
Companion website: www.wiley.com/go/jiyad/handbookofskindiseasemanagement

- **Tirbanibulin ointment** ④: **FT.** The most recently approved therapy for non-hypertrophic AK. Used OD for 5 days. No head-to-head trials to date.
- **Conventional and daylight PDT (cPDT, DL-PDT) with aminolevulinate (ALA) or methyl-ALA** ①: **FT.** Superior to cryotherapy in meta-analyses, but an RCT of 624 participants found treatment success for cPDT was lower than that for 5-FU or imiquimod.
- **Laser resurfacing** ④: **FT.** Ablative or non-ablative fractional lasers are described and may be combined with other topical FTs.
- **Chemical peels** ③: **FT.** In a study of 15, Jessner's + 35% TCA peel reduced visible AKs by 75%, comparable to 5-FU.
- **Systemic chemoprevention:** systemic retinoids and nicotinamide used in chemoprevention of cSCC can also reduce AK burden.

Alopecia areata (AA)

Treatment is largely determined by **age of patient** and **extent of disease** (extensive vs patchy).

Prognosis: ~ 50% with limited patchy hair loss will experience regrowth within a year, but relapse is very common. **Poor prognosis:** severe disease at outset, duration >1 year, atopy and ophiasis pattern.

All Patients

1) Take **baseline photographs.**
2) Recommend **hair camouflage** (see Appendix D)/wigs.

Step 1

- **Potent/superpotent TCS** [2]: use OD. Assess at 3 months and taper gradually.
- **AND/OR IL corticosteroid injections** [3]: 2.5mg/mL as effective as 5–10mg/mL for AA. Injections spaced 1cm apart to affected areas, every 4–6 weeks. Use limited in diffuse disease.
- **Consider oral steroids** [2]: 6-week tapering course encourages *some* degree of regrowth in ~ 75%, but relapse common. Particularly useful in rapidly progressive hair loss.
- **Topical minoxidil** [2]: 5% OD. Generally used *adjunctively*. Use for at least 4 months. Foam preparation has no propylene glycol, which can cause irritation.

Step 2

- **Diphenylcyclopropenone (DPCP)** [3]: see overleaf for application. Use first-line for extensive AA.
- **Squaric acid dibutyl ester (SADBE)** [3]: is alternative if DPCP not available.

Step 3

- **Methotrexate** [3]: 15–25mg alone or in combination with weaning course of oral steroids. A meta-analysis of largely observational studies found a pooled rate of good and complete responses of 63%.

Handbook of Skin Disease Management, First Edition. Zainab Jiyad and Carsten Flohr.
© 2023 John Wiley & Sons Ltd. Published 2023 by John Wiley & Sons Ltd.
Companion website: www.wiley.com/go/jiyad/handbookofskindiseasemanagement

Refractory

- **JAK inhibitors** ③: <u>tofacitinib (5–10mg BD) or baricitinib (4mg/day)</u>, though not widely available. A meta-analysis of cohort studies found a pooled 'good' response of 46%. Evidence suggests hair shedding occurs on discontinuation of tx.
- **Alternatively:** ciclosporin ③, azathioprine ③ (2.5mg/kg), MMF ④.
- **Very limited evidence/availability:** anthralin ④ (<u>see below for application guide</u>), sulfasalazine (<u>0.5g BD build up to 1.5g BD</u>), excimer laser, PUVA, ezetimibe-simvastatin (<u>10mg/40mg</u>).

DPCP application:

- Sensitise with 2% application to small area on non-dominant upper inner arm.
- After 1 week, apply 0.001% solution to alopecia areas.
- Each week, titrate the dose gradually with the aim of achieving low-grade erythema and itching that is tolerable for 1–3 days.
- Titrate as follows: 0.01%, 0.025%, 0.05%, 0.1%, 0.25%, 0.5%, 1%, 2%.
- Most discontinue treatment at 6 months if no response.

Anthralin (dithranol):

- Patient applies 0.5% cream to alopecia areas. Leaves on for 20–30 minutes daily, then rinses off with cool to lukewarm water.
- Aim is to develop 24 hrs of itching/redness.
- Repeat daily.
- Increase time of contact by 10 minutes <u>every 2 weeks, up to 1-hr maximum.</u>
- Thereafter, consider switching to 1% strength, starting at 20 minutes again.

Aphthous ulcers

Differentiate simple vs complex aphthosis, the latter having a history of combined oral and genital ulcers and/or occurring almost continuously.

All Patients

1) **Take a history screening for causes of oral ulceration:** HSV, nutritional deficiencies, SLE, Behcet's, coeliac disease, IBD, HIV, autoimmune bullous disease, neutropenic disorders, lichen planus, fever syndromes, infections, drugs.
2) **Bloods:** FBC, ESR, B12, ferritin, folate. Consider zinc, B2 and B6 as well. Any further tests based on history as above.
3) **Nutritional supplementation:** there is some evidence to suggest B12 supplementation is beneficial, even in the absence of deficiency.

Step 1

Combination of following most effective:
- **Infection/anti-inflammatory** [4]: use chlorhexidine mouthwash BD in all patients and doxycycline dispersible tablet as rinse (100mg dissolved in 10mL water, swish and spit after 2–3 minutes) in most patients. Evidence from RCTs suggests doxycycline reduces number of ulcer days and pain, likely due to anti-inflammatory effects. Avoid in children. Use nystatin suspension QDS in most patients (esp. if using TCS).
- **Analgesia** [4]: lidocaine ointment or spray +/- benzydamine hydrochloride (anti-inflammatory as well) mouthwash/spray every 2–3 hrs.
- **Potent/superpotent TCS** [4]: elixir/gel/ointment availability varies by country (e.g. fluocinolone acetonide gel or fluticasone spray QDS). Alternatively, betamethasone soluble tablets 500 micrograms dissolved in 20 mL of water, swish and spit, QDS. Or fluticasone spray TDS.

Handbook of Skin Disease Management, First Edition. Zainab Jiyad and Carsten Flohr.
© 2023 John Wiley & Sons Ltd. Published 2023 by John Wiley & Sons Ltd.
Companion website: www.wiley.com/go/jiyad/handbookofskindiseasemanagement

Step 2

- **Oral steroids** [4]: short courses for <u>5–7 days of 20–30mg</u>. Not suitable for long-term use.
- **Colchicine** [4]: <u>500 micrograms start at OD and increase to BD after 1 week, as tolerated, to maximum of 2mg</u>. In an RCT comparing with low-dose prednisolone, colchicine was found to be similarly efficacious.
- **Dapsone** [3]: <u>see page 186 for initiation/dosing</u>. Evidence for efficacy in a retrospective review. Can be combined with colchicine in resistant cases.

Refractory

- **Thalidomide** [3]: In a retrospective review of 92,85% underwent complete remission within a median of 14 days. Usually <u>50–100mg/day</u>.
- **Others:** montelukast (RCT vs oral pred = equal), azathioprine, pentoxifylline, levimasole, apremilast, CsA, TNF α-inhibitors.

Atopic dermatitis (AD)

Treatment of atopic dermatitis requires good support and engagement with parents. Age must be factored in – the algorithm below *pertains to children 5 years and over/adults.* For management in younger ages, see overleaf.

All Patients

1) Establish diagnosis and **severity/extent of the disease.** In routine clinical practice POEM score or Patient Global Assessment (PGA) is sufficient. EASI/ SCORAD or other physician-assessed scores are mainly used in research settings.
2) Assess impact on **quality of life (DLQI/CDLQI), sleep, and psychological well-being,** including impact on the whole family.
3) Direct parents/patients to various **information sources** available: https:// eczema.org/ (National Eczema Society) and https://www.eos.org.uk/ (Eczema Outreach Support), and British Association of Dermatologists patient information leaflets; habit reversal to address the itch–scratch cycle: https://www.atopicskindisease.com/.
4) Nurse-led eczema education session, if available

Step 1

- **Moisturiser** ①: regular and liberal emollient application cannot be overemphasised. Use preparation that works best for patient/parents and ensures compliance. ~250–500 grams per week in someone with widespread AD/dry skin.
- **Soap substitute** ①: many select one with antibacterial properties (e.g. Dermol 500® lotion), but in general any emollient will suffice as soap substitute. Aqueous cream should be avoided, as it can cause skin irritation.
- **TCS** ①: *OD application equivalent efficacy to BD. Use ointments preferably.* Start with low–medium potency, escalate to medium-potent if poor response. Advise weaning TCS, rather than abrupt stop. Consider twice weekly treatment for maintenance.
- **Topical pimecrolimus and tacrolimus** ①: useful as steroid alternative, often most helpful for maintenance treatment and in areas with higher risk of skin thinning. Tacrolimus 0.1% has potent anti-inflammatory effect (vs tacrolimus 0.03% and pimecrolimus 1%, which have low potency).

Handbook of Skin Disease Management, First Edition. Zainab Jiyad and Carsten Flohr.
© 2023 John Wiley & Sons Ltd. Published 2023 by John Wiley & Sons Ltd.
Companion website: www.wiley.com/go/jiyad/handbookofskindiseasemanagement

Step 2

- **Phototherapy** [2]: NBUVB is generally preferred. An SR concluded preference of UVA1 and NBUVB.
- **Methotrexate** [3]: generally used as systemic of choice, although a network MA suggested less efficacy than ciclosporin and azathioprine. *See page 181 for initiation and dose.*
- **Ciclosporin** [3]: Second-line systemic. *See page 183 for dosing.* Often used where acute control needed.
- **Dupilumab** [3]: A meta-analysis of RCTs has shown superiority over other systemics – some believe this should be used first-line. UK NICE guidelines recommend using only if another systemic (CsA/MTX/AZA/MMF) has failed or cannot be given. At 16 weeks, EASI 50 should be achieved (50% reduction EASI score) and 4-point reduction in DLQI. *See page 197 for dosing.*
- **Others:** azathioprine and MMF are also used, though increasingly less frequently. *See page 185 and 188 for initiation and dosing.*

Infants & <5 years

- Above algorithm also applies.
- Bandages or stockinette garments/wet wraps can be useful, especially when AD is widespread. Their application will need parent education at the outset, see https://www.stjohnsdermacademy.com/patient-resources for video demonstration.
- In infants with severe AD/other systemic symptoms, such as failure to thrive and recurrent deep-seated infections, consider immunodeficiencies, such as hyper-IgE and Netherton syndrome.

Other key management points

- **JAK inhibitors: abrocitinib/baracitinib/upadacitinib** are now NICE approved for AD and increasingly used, particularly when dupilumab has failed or is contraindicated.
- **Crisaborole:** a topical PDE4 inhibitor. A network meta-analysis suggested comparable efficacy to mild potency TCS. Not available in the UK/Europe.
- **Oral corticosteroids:** acute exacerbations are often treated with weaning courses of oral steroids as rescue therapy, *e.g. 30mg reduce (~0.5mg/kg/day) by 5mg each week then stop.* Only use if severe flare, for instance due to skin infection. Avoid frequent courses or long-term treatment.
- **Managing infection:** Staph. aureus colonisation is almost universal in atopic dermatitis. If there are recurrent infections, swabbing and eradicating staph. carriage may help, including from the nose with antibiotic nasal ointment. Most infections can be treated topically, but oral antibiotics are indicated if widespread or severe.
- **Diluted bleach baths:** although widely practiced (twice weekly) and recommended, a meta-analysis found no superiority over bathing in plain water.

Food allergies: who, what, and when to test

- **What are the types of food allergy?** 2 main categories: **1)** IgE-mediated (immediate, usually within 2 hrs post-food ingestion) that presents with urticaria, lip and facial swelling (angioedema), wheezing, and GI symptoms (nausea, diarrhoea) and, if severe, anaphylaxis (main foods: cow's milk, egg, wheat, cod fish, sesame, peanut, and soya); **2)** non-IgE-mediated reactions (delayed symptoms, usually within 24 hrs): flare of AD but also reflux and abdominal pain/diarrhoea; main foods: cow's milk, egg, wheat, soya.
- **How common is food-exacerbated atopic dermatitis?** Food *sensitisation* is common and does not equate to a food allergy. The prevalence of food allergy is low in those with mild AD and rises to almost a third in moderate-to-severe AD. It is rare in adults, especially new-onset food allergy.
- **Do elimination diets work for AD?** A Cochrane meta-analysis concluded there was little evidence for exclusion diets in *unselected populations*. However, a careful allergy history for both immediate and delayed reactions to foods needs to be taken in all children with AD and investigated accordingly. Where in doubt, referral to a (paediatric) allergist should be considered as well as a (paediatric) dietitian, in case of food exclusions.
- **Who should be tested?** Anyone with suggestive hx. Broad allergy panel testing without a history suggestive of an allergy should be avoided, although a negative test result can be helpful when parents/patients are convinced that the AD is caused by foods. *See chart overleaf.*
- **Which tests?** Most dermatologists start with specific IgE testing on blood (ImmunoCAP), before skin-prick testing. Both will only detect IgE-mediated allergy – if high suspicion and negative test, consider 4–6-week trial of dietary exclusion (suspicion of non-IgE mediated hypersensitivity) or food challenge via a paediatric allergy team. *See chart below for testing algorithm.*

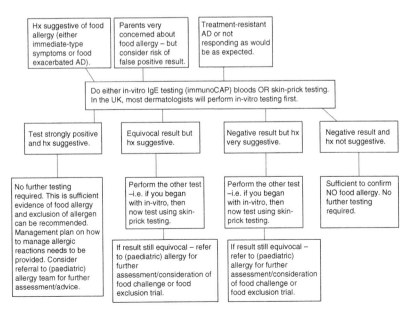

Algorithm: Testing for food allergy in atopic dermatitis.

Basal cell carcinoma (BCC)

BCC has a very small risk of metastasising, hence traditional cancer staging is rarely applied. Rather, BCC is stratified into **high risk** and **low risk** of recurrence, as per the table below.

Criteria for low-risk and high-risk basal cell carcinoma (BCC)

Parameters	Low risk	High risk
Clinical criteria		
Location/size	Area L ≤ 20mm* Area M ≤ 10mm**	Area L > 20mm* Area M > 10mm** All area H***
Borders	Well defined	Poorly defined
Primary vs. recurrent	Primary	Recurrent
Immunosuppression	No	Yes
Site of prior radiotherapy	No	Yes
Pathological criteria		
Growth pattern	Nodular or superficial	Infiltrative (infiltrating, morphoeic, micronodular)
Differentiation: basosquamous	Absent	Present
Level of invasion	Dermis, subcutaneous fat	Beyond subcutaneous fat
Depth (thickness)	≤ 6mm	> 6mm
Perineural invasion (named nerve or diameter ≥ 0.1mm or beyond the dermis)	Absent	Present
TNM stage	pT1 ≤ 20mm	pT2 >20 mm but ≤40 mm; pT3 >40 mm, or upstaged pT1 or pT2, or minor bone invasion; pT4 major bone invasion
Margins		
Histological margins	Not involved (≥ 1mm)	Involved or histologically close (< 1mm)

*L area: trunk and extremities (excluding those in H areas below).

**M area: cheeks, forehead, scalp, neck, and pretibial area. See figure below.

***H area: central face, eyelids, eyebrows, periorbital skin, nose, lips, chin, mandible, preauricular and postauricular skin, temple, ear, genitalia, hands, and feet. See figure below

Handbook of Skin Disease Management, First Edition. Zainab Jiyad and Carsten Flohr.
© 2023 John Wiley & Sons Ltd. Published 2023 by John Wiley & Sons Ltd.
Companion website: www.wiley.com/go/jiyad/handbookofskindiseasemanagement

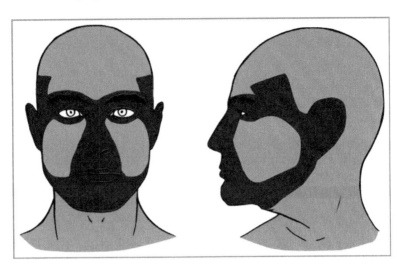

Areas H (darker shade) and M (lighter shade) on the head and neck. *Source:* Nasr I, McGrath EJ, Harwood CA, et al. British Association of Dermatologists guidelines for the management of adults with basal cell carcinoma 2021. Br J Dermatol 2021;185(5):899–920.

> **Low-risk options**
>
> - **Surgical excision** ①: studies have shown this to be superior to other treatments. *Generally considered first-line*, although many prefer topical treatment or destructive therapy for pure superficial BCC subtypes. UK guidelines: 4–5mm margins; AAD guidelines: 4mm margins; European guidelines: 3–4mm margins.
> - **Imiquimod** ①: daily for 5 nights of each week for 6 weeks for superficial BCC. RCT vs surgery found 3-year cure rates to be 85% for imiquimod group vs 98% for excision. Meta-analysis estimated 14.1% recurrence rate.
> - **5-FU** ①: in RCT of 601 participants, 5-year tumor-free survival was 70% for 5-FU (63% for PDT and 81% for imiquimod). Meta-analysis estimated 18.8% recurrence rate.
> - **PDT** ①: in a network meta-analysis, estimated recurrence rate was 18.8% with MAL-PDT.
> - **Cryotherapy** ③: use is largely limited to superficial BCCs, but the recurrence rate is high – 22.3% in meta-analysis.
> - **Radiotherapy** ③: generally reserved for high-risk BCCs, see below.
> - **Curettage and cautery** ③: a non-randomised trial reported 5-year recurrence rates ranging from 1.2% (best-case scenario) to 20.6% (where losses to follow-up considered recurrences). Higher rates reported in high-risk BCCs.

- **Mohs micrographic surgery (MMS)** [4]: *treatment of choice.* Randomised study comparing MMS with standard excision found recurrence rates to be 2.5% vs 4.1% (at 5 years) and 4.4% vs 12.2% (at 10 years).

- **Standard excision** [3]: as above. This is an alternative treatment where MMS is not available. **Staged excision ('slow Mohs')** is another option. European guidelines recommend 5-15mm margin for high-risk BCCs where MMS not possible.

- **Radiotherapy** [3]: where surgery is not feasible, this is the preferred second-line treatment. Its non-invasive nature makes it an appealing option, particularly in elderly patients. In one RCT of radiotherapy vs surgery, 4-year recurrence rate was 7.5% vs 0.7%. In meta-analysis estimated recurrence rate was 3.5%.

- **PDT** [3]: in a study of 102 patients with high-risk BCCs, the 2-year complete response rate was 78%.

- **Destructive/topical treatments as per low risk (previous page):** only where above treatments not feasible.

Behçet's Disease

This should be diagnosed by a multidisciplinary team including a range of relevant specialists. The mucocutaneous manifestations of Behçet's are the most common presentation of the disease, but any organ can be involved, resulting in various manifestations requiring specific management by the relevant specialist in the Behçet's team. The most commonly used diagnostic criteria are below. Unlike the ISG, the ICBD does not stress the need for oral ulceration in making the diagnosis. Lesions may occur acutely in any organ resulting in end organ damage, and this requires prompt immunosuppression to prevent morbidity and mortality.

International Criteria for Behçet's Disease (ICBD) – point score system: scoring ≥4 indicates Behçet's diagnosis:

Signs/symptoms	Points
Ocular lesions	2
Genital aphthosis	2
Oral aphthosis	2
Skin lesions	1
Neurological manifestations	1
Vascular manifestations	1
Positive pathergy test (optional)	1

International Study Group (ISG) for Behçet's Disease:

Essential	
Recurrent oral ulceration	Observed by clinician or patient, with at least three episodes in any 12-month period.
Plus any two of following:	
Recurrent genital ulceration	Observed by clinician or patient; look for evidence of scarring on the affected surface.
Eye lesions	Anterior or posterior uveitis cells in vitreous on slit-lamp examination, or retinal vasculitis; retinal vein thrombosis.
Skin lesions	Erythema nodosum-like lesions observed by clinician or patient; papulopustular skin lesions or pseudofolliculitis with characteristic acneiform nodules observed by clinician.
Gastrointestinal lesions	Ulceration.

Handbook of Skin Disease Management, First Edition. Zainab Jiyad and Carsten Flohr.
© 2023 John Wiley & Sons Ltd. Published 2023 by John Wiley & Sons Ltd.
Companion website: www.wiley.com/go/jiyad/handbookofskindiseasemanagement

Treat the different mucocutaneous manifestations of Behcet's on merit:

Oral ulceration	• See aphthous ulcers page 12, step 1 ONLY, + topical sucrulfate (below).
Vasculitis	• Manage as per vasculitis section, see page 172.
Erythema nodosum	• Manage as per erythema nodosum section, see page 55.
Pyoderma gangrenosum	• Manage as per PG section, see page 149.
Other cutaneous/genital ulcers	• Manage as below.

Cutaneous

Skin lesions in Behcet's:

- **Potent/superpotent TCS** [4]: OD/BD.
- **Colchicine** [2]: widely used after in conjunction with TCS. Use <u>500 micrograms start at OD and increase to BD after 1 week, as tolerated, to maximum of 2mg</u>.
- **Others:** azathioprine or biological agents may be indicated in more severe disease.

Genital ulcers

- **Topical steroids** [4]: potent commonly used. <u>OD/BD</u>.
- **Topical calcineurin inhibitors** [2]: placebo-controlled RCT of 90 found <u>pimecrolimus BD</u> significantly reduced healing time.
- **Colchicine** [2]: used in conjunction with TCS. Placebo-controlled RCT of 116 found a significant reduction in the mean number of genital ulcers in the treated group (0.1 vs 2.6). <u>Dose as above</u>.
- **Azathioprine** [2]: a placebo-controlled RCT found a significant reduction in number of genital ulcers at 24 months. Standard dosing, see page 185.
- **Dapsone** [2]: placebo crossover study of 20 found significant reduction of genital ulcers in dapsone group. Standard dosing, see page 186.
- **Others:** etanercept, apremilast, depot steroid injections.

Bowen's disease (SCC in-situ)

The risk of Bowen's progressing to invasive SCC is estimated at around 3–5%. The **choice of treatment** depends on the site (cosmetically sensitive, poor healing), ability to commit to course of treatment (PDT, 5-FU), and patient preference.

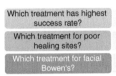

Which treatment has highest success rate?	• Highest success rates with PDT. Excision also very successful
Which treatment for poor healing sites?	• Sites such as lower limbs, ideally use PDT. Avoid cryotherapy, surgery and radiotherapy
Which treatment for facial Bowen's?	• Curettage commonly used. PDT, 5-FU, imiquimod very reasonable options too

5-FU

② Variable regimens, but higher success rates reported with intense/longer courses. <u>Use BD for 3–8 weeks, as tolerated.</u> In RCT of 225, 5-FU vs PDT vs cryotherapy, complete response rates at 3 months were 83% vs 93% and 86%, respectively.

Imiquimod

② In a placebo-controlled RCT of 31, 11 of 15 treated achieved resolution (73%). <u>Use OD for up to 16 weeks, usually at least 6 weeks of treatment required.</u>

C&C

③ Reported recurrence rates vary from 2 to 20%. In a study of 67 patients of curettage vs cryotherapy, healing time and recurrence rates were both better with curettage.

PDT

① As per study above, reported clearance rates at 3 months of 93%. Sustained clearance rates after 2 years are lower but generally around 70% or higher.

Cryotherapy

② Rapid treatment makes this an attractive and widely used treatment option. Avoid on the lower leg. Variable recurrence rates and clearance rates reported, reflecting different cryotherapy regimens.

Others

- **Excision** ③: uncommonly used, consider excision margins of 4–6 mm.
- **Radiotherapy** ③: rarely used and no standardised protocol.
- **Laser** ③: rarely used. In a study of 44, × 1 treatment with CO_2 laser cleared 86%. Consider for digits/genitalia.

Handbook of Skin Disease Management, First Edition. Zainab Jiyad and Carsten Flohr.
© 2023 John Wiley & Sons Ltd. Published 2023 by John Wiley & Sons Ltd.
Companion website: www.wiley.com/go/jiyad/handbookofskindiseasemanagement

Bullous pemphigoid

Treatment depends on extent of disease (localised vs generalised) and patient's abilities to manage topicals/monitoring of systemics. In those with moderate-severe disease, progress straight to oral steroids, whilst using topicals adjunctively.

All Patients

1) **Check drugs – causation link weak in most:** gliptins, furosemide, amlodipine, ACE inhibitors, NSAIDs, gabapentin, others.
2) **Take a skin biopsy for histology (lesional skin) and direct immunofluorescence (IMF) (perilesional skin):** *see page 218.* Some advocate testing serum for indirect immunofluorescence as well. Screening bloods for systemics initiation usually performed at diagnosis.
3) **Recommend good skin care as follows:** deflate blisters with sterile needle and leave blister roof on; wash with antibacterial lotion; regular use of barrier ointment; non-adhesive dressings.

Step 1

- **Superpotent TCS** [4]: often prescribed BD but OD increasingly used and likely equally efficacious. In a RCT of 341, found to be superior to oral steroids on several parameters including safety profile and speed to response. However, most would still use oral steroids in addition for moderate–severe disease.

Step 2

- **Oral steroids** [4]: prednisolone 0.5–1mg/kg/day, as a gradual weaning regimen. *See page 129 for tapering guide.*
- **AND tetracyclines** [4]: doxycycline 100mg BD. BLISTER trial compared it to prednisolone and found it to be non-inferior, but in clinical practice tetracyclines rarely produce rapid and effective control as sole agent.

Handbook of Skin Disease Management, First Edition. Zainab Jiyad and Carsten Flohr.
© 2023 John Wiley & Sons Ltd. Published 2023 by John Wiley & Sons Ltd.
Companion website: www.wiley.com/go/jiyad/handbookofskindiseasemanagement

Step 3

Steroid-sparing agents are often initiated whilst oral steroids are slowly tapered to prevent flare:

- **MMF** ④: equally as efficacious as azathioprine in RCT of 73. See page 188 for dosing.
- **Azathioprine** ④: *most commonly used.* See page 185 for dosing.
- **Methotrexate** ③: review of uncontrolled studies – 74 of 79 improved. Increasingly favored due to low side effects. See page 181 for initiation and dosing.

Refractory

- **Dapsone** ②: in a review of the literature, 139 of 170 patients showed improvement (with/without other agents). Regular blood monitoring required makes it an unpractical choice for elderly patients. See page 186 for initiation and dosing.
- **Others** ②: **rituximab vs omalizumab** – although SR found similar response rates (85% vs 84%), rituximab recurrence rate was much lower (29% vs 80%). **IVIG –** a review of 45 patients reported 86% improved.
- **Rarely used** ④: ciclosporin, cyclophosphamide, chlorambucil, dupilumab.

Calciphylaxis

Whilst the majority of cases relate to end-stage renal failure, *non-uraemic calciphylaxis* is a recognised entity with obesity, diabetes, malignancies, autoimmune diseases, primary hyperparathyroidism and alcoholic liver disease being the main causes.

All Patients

1) **Analgesia:** pain is the hallmark of calciphylaxis. Ensure appropriate analgesia, involve pain team as necessary.
2) **Good wound care:** specialist nursing care is imperative, particularly as sepsis from wounds is the main cause of mortality in calciphylaxis. Debridement is debatable, but most agree that debridement should be considered for infected necrotic wounds.
3) **Manage key risk factors:** stop calcium, calcium-containing phosphate binders, and vitamin D supplementation; stop warfarin; manage obesity and diabetes, which impact on both uraemic and non-uraemic calciphylaxis.

Step 1

- **Sodium thiosulphate (STS)** [3]: in a retrospective review of 53, 26% completely resolved and just under 50% improved; though a meta-analysis of retrospective studies did not find benefit for any treatments, including STS in calciphylaxis. Normally introduced at 5g 3 times a week and then uptitrated to 25g 3 times a week (or 12.5g if weight <60kg). Given IV during the last 30–60 minutes of hemodialysis, usually continued for 3 months.

Step 2

- **Cinacalcet** [3]: extremes of PTH level should be avoided (too high/too low). In RCT of 3500 treated with cinacalcet, there was a reduced incidence of calciphylaxis in the treated group. But the evidence for improving calciphylaxis is less robust. Should be initiated by the renal team.
- **Bisphosphonates** [3]: some evidence of success from case reports/retrospective studies. Meta-analysis (non-RCTs) showed no benefit, e.g. disodium pamidronate 30mg IV monthly.

Handbook of Skin Disease Management, First Edition. Zainab Jiyad and Carsten Flohr.
© 2023 John Wiley & Sons Ltd. Published 2023 by John Wiley & Sons Ltd.
Companion website: www.wiley.com/go/jiyad/handbookofskindiseasemanagement

Refractory

- **Anticoagulation** [4]: warfarin exacerbates calciphylaxis. Part of the aetiology of calciphlaxis is believed to be hypercoagulability, and there are case reports of success with heparin. <u>Use tinzaparin treatment-dose or unfractionated heparin. Apixaban may be considered in some cases.</u>

- **Increase dialysis/kidney transplantation** [3]: transplantation may not be an option for many patients. The benefit of intensifying dialysis is conflicting, with one study finding an increased risk of death with intensified regimen.

Central centrifugal cicatricial alopecia (CCCA)

As with all scarring alopecias, explain that the **aim** is to treat active disease to prevent further hair loss and that scarred, 'burnt out' areas will not be reversible. Encourage early treatment to prevent irreversible progression.

Active disease is suggested by:

- Symptoms (itching, pain, burning, etc.).
- Inflammation (erythema, papules, etc.).
- Ongoing hair loss.
- Active disease on biopsy.

All Patients

1) **Behavioural modifications:** stop chemical relaxers, avoid excessive traction. See Appendix D (afro-hair tips).
2) **Consider biopsy** (see page 217).
3) Take **baseline photographs.**
4) Recommend **hair camouflage** (see Appendix D)/wigs.

At any stage consider tapering course of **oral steroids** (0.5–1mg/kg) to stabilise active disease.

Step 1

- **Potent/superpotent TCS** [4]: use OD to active areas, assess at 3 month and taper gradually.
- **AND/OR IL corticosteroid injections** [4]: 10mg/mL (reduce to 5mg/mL for frontal scalp), to edge of active areas.
- **Topical minoxidil** [4]: use 5%. Consider a trial of this for at least 4 months to assess efficacy. Explain this would only influence undamaged hair follicles. Foam preparation has no propylene glycol, which can cause irritation (especially in inflamed scalp).
- Treat any concurrent **androgenetic alopecia.**

Handbook of Skin Disease Management, First Edition. Zainab Jiyad and Carsten Flohr.
© 2023 John Wiley & Sons Ltd. Published 2023 by John Wiley & Sons Ltd.
Companion website: www.wiley.com/go/jiyad/handbookofskindiseasemanagement

Step 2

- **Tetracyclines** [4]: All patients except those with very mild disease should be initiated on <u>doxycycline 100mg OD/BD</u>. Continue for 3 months and very gradually reduce once inflammation settles. Based on expert opinion.

Step 3

- **Hydroxychloroquine** [4]: <u>200mg BD or OD (max 5mg/kg)</u>. Based on expert opinion.

Refractory

- **Consider:** MMF, ciclosporin.

Chilblains (perniosis)

With COVID-19, perniosis has become a widely recognised disease. It is important to be aware that there are other cold-induced dermatoses as well as secondary causes of perniosis, such as haematological disorders.

All Patients

1) Take a **history screening for other cold-associated conditions** that can be confused with perniosis: see page 203 for full list. COVID-19 is also associated with perniosis.
2) If the hx and clinical signs are strongly suggestive of idiopathic chilblains, no further testing is usually required. Otherwise, **perform the following Ix:** punch bx + IMF, FBC, U/Es, protein electrophoresis, immunoglobulins, ANA, cryoglobulins, cold agglutinins, cryofibrinogens.

Step 1

- **Cold avoidance and insulating clothing** [4]: recommend thermal gloves/socks.
- **TCS** [2]: the evidence for efficacy is poor – a placebo-controlled RCT of 34 showed no difference. However, they are frequently trialled first-line.

Step 2

- **Nifedipine** [2]: RCT of nifedipine vs diltiazem – 21/24 in nifedipine group showed 80–90% improvement vs only 5/12 in diltiazem group. Start with 5mg TDS and increase to 10mg TDS as tolerated.

Step 3

- **Pentoxifylline** [2]: in a placebo-controlled RCT of 118, 40/55 (73%) in the pentoxifylline group achieved a very good response at 3 weeks compared with 11/55 (20%) in placebo arm. Use 400mg TDS.
- **Diltiazem** [2]: in above RCT vs nifedipine, less than half improved. Use 60mg TDS.

Refractory

- **Topical minoxidil/GTN** [2]: both topical minoxidil and topical GTN have been compared with nifedipine in trials and showed less benefit, but as they are topicals and have minimal side effects, can consider a trial early on in treatment.
- **Others:** topical tacrolimus, nicotinamide.

Handbook of Skin Disease Management, First Edition. Zainab Jiyad and Carsten Flohr.
© 2023 John Wiley & Sons Ltd. Published 2023 by John Wiley & Sons Ltd.
Companion website: www.wiley.com/go/jiyad/handbookofskindiseasemanagement

Chondrodermatitis nodularis helicis

Whilst some proceed with surgery at the outset due to the relatively high recurrence rates we recommend topicals here before surgery.

Step 1

- **Pressure relief** [2]: different methods used including self-adhering foam, foam bandages, or doughnut-shaped pillows. A SR concluded cure rates of 37% for pressure relief alone, based on 5 studies. However, recurrence rates are reported at around 30%.
- **Topicals corticosteroids** [3]: the above SR reported cure rates of 35% from 2 studies.
- **IL steroids** [3]: 2–10mg/mL injections of triamcinalone can be beneficial. In a study of 60, the reported response rate was 60%.
- **Topical nitroglycerin (UK = glyceryl trinitrate)** [3]: available as 0.4% ointment. Higher concentrations need compounding and may be unstable. Reported overall cure rate of 27%. Use BD for up to 8 weeks. Headache is a side effect.

Step 2

- **Surgery** [3]: various methods have been used including wedge excision and wide excision with flaps/grafts. Broadly, techniques can be divided into excision of both cartilage and skin vs cartilage only.

  Recurrences tend to occur at the edges of the cartilage defect, so meticulous trimming is advised. Overall cure rate 82%.

Refractory

- **Laser** [3]: studies based on CO_2 laser and argon laser report cure rates ranging from 56 to 100%.
- **PDT** [4]: in a series of 5, the reported cure rate was 80%.
- **Others:** bacitracin ointment, cryotherapy, collagen injections, procaine injections, platelet-rich plasma.

Chronic actinic dermatitis (CAD)

Differentiating photosensitivity from photoaggravated disorders is important clinically, *see page 207 & 208 for list of causes*. A punch biopsy may be undertaken in CAD – a differential to consider is CTCL, especially if erythrodermic.

All Patients

1) **Patch testing and photopatch testing:** usually performed. The former is required due to the high prevalence of allergic contact dermatitis in patients with CAD. Photopatch testing may be indicated to rule out concurrent sunscreen allergy.
2) **Blood screen for lupus:** *see page 103 for list*. Not always necessary. Test for HIV if any risk factor/concerns.
3) **Advise careful photoprotection:** behaviour, clothes, hats, appropriate high SPF sunscreen use.
4) **Vitamin D supplementation.**

Course of oral corticosteroids can be used for severe or acute flares, e.g. 20–40mg as reducing regimen over 6 weeks.

Step 1

- **Topical corticosteroids** [4]: variable potencies used, depending on site. Used first-line, OD/BD.
- **Topical calcineurin inhibitors** [4]: reports/series showing success. Use OD/BD.

Step 2

- **Azathioprine** [2]: in a placebo-controlled RCT of 18, 5 of 8 treated with azathioprine achieved complete remission on clinical assessment vs none in the placebo group. Use standard dosing, see page 185.
- **Ciclosporin** [4]: reports/series of success. Use standard dosing, see page 183.
- **MMF** [4]: case reports of success. Use standard dosing, see page 188.
- **Methotrexate** [4]: case series of success.
- **Dupilumab** [4]: case series of success.
- **PUVA** [4]: case series of success.

Handbook of Skin Disease Management, First Edition. Zainab Jiyad and Carsten Flohr.
© 2023 John Wiley & Sons Ltd. Published 2023 by John Wiley & Sons Ltd.
Companion website: www.wiley.com/go/jiyad/handbookofskindiseasemanagement

Contact dermatitis

> **When to consider patch testing:**
> - Suspected contact dermatitis.
> - Atopic eczema where an additional contact allergy is suspected or in poorly controlled eczema.
> - Eczema: hand/foot, facial, ano-genital, varicose; otitis externa.
> - Consider clothing dermatitis with peri-axillary, waistband, inner thighs eczema or under a bandage/support stocking.

> **Patch test grading: –** No reaction;
> **?** = doubtful reaction; irritant reaction (no infiltration; wrinkling; reaction within chamber).
> **+** Weak reaction with erythema, infiltration, and papules.
> **++** Strong reaction: vesicles, erythema, infiltration, papules.
> **+++** Spreading bullous reaction.

Allergens from Extended European Standard Battery	
Metals	
Nickel sulfate	Metal objects such as jewellery, fasteners, jeans studs, coins (generally only relevant if working with money), glasses, artificial joints, eyelash curlers, dental braces. Co-sensitivity with cobalt. Use the dimethylglyoxime test (pink= +ve).
Potassium dichromate	Used in tanning of leather and commonest cause of shoe allergy; wet concrete, paints, orthopedic and dental implants, cosmetics.
Cobalt chloride	See nickel list; also cement, paint, ceramics, vitamin B12 (can cause cheilitis from oral vitamin B12 and dermatitis from parenteral use).

> **Nickel, cobalt, and chromate allergy are associated with implant loosening and failure in metal-on-metal arthroplasties. Recommend patch testing if history of metal allergy and if positive, avoid prostheses with these metals.**
> **Nickel and cobalt can be found as contaminants (i.e. not listed in ingredients) in eye make-up; do repeated open application test to investigate (see below).**

Handbook of Skin Disease Management, First Edition. Zainab Jiyad and Carsten Flohr.
© 2023 John Wiley & Sons Ltd. Published 2023 by John Wiley & Sons Ltd.
Companion website: www.wiley.com/go/jiyad/handbookofskindiseasemanagement

Preservatives: Cosmetics, skin and hair care products, soaps/cleansers, sunscreens, baby wipes, paints, laundry products, deodorants	
Formaldehyde	Widely used preservative. Also found in household products, textiles.
Quaternium-15	Formaldehyde releaser, medicated shampoos, some prescribed creams.
Imidazolidinyl urea	Formaldehyde releaser.
Diazolidinyl urea	Formaldehyde releaser.
2-Bromo-2-nitropropane-1,3-diol (bronopol)	Formaldehyde releaser, antimicrobial used as a preservative.
Paraben mix	Can also be in prescribed creams.
Methylchloroisothiazolinone/ methylisothiazolinone	Paints (can cause an airborne dermatitis), ask about decorating; ironing water. Now banned from leave-on products.
Methyldibromo glutaronitrile	Detergents and washing-up liquids, ultrasound gel, glues, and paints. Banned in leave-on and wash-off products.
Octylisothiazolinone Benzisothiazolinone	Fungicides and bactericides used in leather products, cosmetics, and shampoos. Laundry products – may rarely cause an allergy. Paints, sealants.
Fragrances: perfumes and aftershaves, lotions/creams, cosmetics, laundry products, household cleaning products, toothpaste and mouthwash, bath products, air fresheners. Advise patients to avoid products containing 'parfum', 'perfume', 'fragrance', or 'aroma'	
Fragrance mix I	= cinnamic alcohol, cinnamic aldehyde, hydroxycitronellal, amylcinnamaldehyde, geraniol, euginol, isoeuginol, oakmoss absolute.
Fragrance mix II	= lyral, citral, citronellol, farnesol, coumarin, hexyl cinnamic aldehyde.
Myroxylon pereirae (balsam of Peru)	Natural mixture of plants, chemicals, and essential oils found in cough mixtures, eugenol, Chinese balms. Can act as an antiseptic and is found in Anusol® (which can cause initial sensitisation). May react to spices such as cinnamon, cloves, cardamom, and nutmeg as well as citrus fruit peel and chewing gum.
Hydroxyisohexyl 3-cyclohexene carboxaldehyde (Lyral)	Synthetic fragrance also known as Lyral or HICC.
Rubber	
Thiuram mix 2-Mercaptobenzothiazole (MBT)	Rubber accelerator, found in rubber gloves, elastic, condoms, tubular bandages, rubber soles, adhesives.

N-isopropyl-N-phenyl-para-phenylenediamine (IPPD)	Antioxidant in rubber production found in black rubber products, e.g. black rubber boots, tyres, wetsuits. May cross react with PPD.
Mercapto mix	See thiuram mix. Most frequently used rubber accelerator in shoes or insoles and old shoes may be more allergenic.

Topical medication

Neomycin sulphate	Topical antibiotic (may also have an allergy to gentamicin and framycetin). Eye drops, ear drops/sprays, e.g. Otomize®, topical antibiotics, creams, e.g. Betnovate N®, Naseptin®
Caine mix	Benzocaine, amethocaine, cinochocaine. Topical anaesthetic creams, lozenges, cough spray. Lignocaine is safe. May cross react with PPD and azo dyes.

Steroids: if positive do the full steroid battery. Late positives are common.

Budesonide	(Group B and some Group D corticosteroids.) Useful marker for steroid allergy. Found in asthma inhalers and nasal sprays
Tixocortol pivalate	Marker for hydrocortisone (Group A corticosteroids). Found in many creams, hemorrhoid preparations, etc.

Adhesives

Epoxy resin (bisphenol A)	Found in 2-part glues, e.g. Araldite® (usually not allergenic once hardened). Can cause hand eczema and an airborne dermatitis. Also causes allergies in industry.
Colophonium (colophony)	Plasters, cosmetics, hair-removing wax, dental products, glues and adhesives, varnishes, rosin for musical strings, racket grips.
Para-Tertiary-butylphenol-formaldehyde resin (PTBP resin)	Leather/rubber adhesives (e.g. shoes, watch straps); lacquers, varnishes.

Plants

Sesquiterpene lactone mix	Indicates an allergy to Compositae group of plants. Creams and lotions, cosmetics. May cause hand eczema or airborne dermatitis. Common allergy seen in patients with chronic actinic dermatitis.
Compositae mix	Sesquiterpene lactose mix/Compositae mix.

Dyes

Textile dye mix	A mixture of disperse dyes, which are the most common sensitisers. Fabric dyes, avoid synthetic fabrics and wash new clothes before wearing.
p-phenylenediamine free base (PPD)	Found in all semi-permanent and permanent hair dyes (dye only allergenic when wet). PPD may be added to black henna tattoos, inducing allergy. Can cause a clothing dye allergy. If history of severe allergy, reduce concentration or do short exposure when patch testing.

Others	
Sodium metabisulphate	Sulphites used as antioxidants. Found in creams, e.g. Trimovate®, Timodine®, Nizoral®. Also found in fresh fruits to prevent browning and wine/beer and can cause a systemic reaction if ingested.
Propolis	A mixture of essential oils, resins, and waxes, collected by bees. Lip balm, cough syrup, toothpaste, creams, and shampoos.
Wool alcohols (Amerchol and lanolin)	Hand lotions, moisturisers, sunscreen, cosmetics, furniture polishes, leather, lubricants, some medicaments (Synalar®, Fucidin®).
Decyl glucoside	Surfactant in body washes, shampoos, skin-care products.
Lauryl glucoside	See decyl glucoside.
Cetearyl alcohol	In many creams (including steroid and anti-infection creams) and a few ointments; hair conditioner.
2-hydroxyethyl methacrylate (HEMA)	Artificial (heat-cured) nails, dental materials, lacquers. Can cause an airborne dermatitis.

Repeated open application test (ROAT):
Patients can test their own products by applying them twice a day for 2 weeks to the same site on their forearms and seeing if they develop a reaction.

Testing patients' products:
Patients' products can be tested including clothing; *wash-off products need to be diluted.*

Patch testing children:
The prevalence of allergic contact dermatitis in children is increasing. Consider patch testing children aged 6 or above where the history/examination is suggestive or if eczema is resistant to treatment. An adapted battery is used for children.

Darier disease

A number of clinical variants of Darier disease have been described including hypotrophic, intertriginous and segmental. Segmental subtype is particularly amenable to interventional therapies. Darier disease can be associated with neuropsychiatric conditions and a two-fold increased risk of diabetes.

All Patients

1) Measures to **avoid sweating (keep skin cool).**
2) Recommend chlorhexidine or other **antimicrobial wash.**
3) **Treat maladour and secondary infection** intermittently as required with topical/oral antibiotics.
4) **There is a high rate of HSV:** swab and treat with aciclovir if suspected or proven.

Step 1

- **Moderately potent–potent TCS** [4]: use OD/BD. Use the lowest potency that is effective.
- **Topical retinoids** [4]: may cause irritation, so consider alternate-day application. Can also use in combination with TCS to lessen irritation. Use adapelene, tretinoin 0.1%, or tazoretene OD.
- **Topical antibiotics** [4]: superinfection is not uncommon, and intermittent treatment can be beneficial. Clindamycin, mupirocin often used.

Step 2

- **Acitretin** [3]: most commonly used systemic. In a double-blind study of acitretin vs etretinate, 10 of 13 treated with 30mg of acitretin improved. Standard dosing, see Appendix A.
- **Isotretinoin** [3]: alternative to acitretin. Typically doses of 0.5–1mg/kg, Appendix A.
- **Alitretinoin (less commonly used)** [4]: evidence from case reports. Standard dosing, see Appendix A.

Refractory

- **Naltrexone** [3]: 5mg OD has been reported to show benefit in small case series.
- **Interventional** [4]: lasers, surgical excision, dermabrasion, PDT, Botox, electron beam radiation.
- **Others** [4]: topical tacrolimus, 5-FU, diclofenac sodium 3% gel, topical glycopyrrolate.

Handbook of Skin Disease Management, First Edition. Zainab Jiyad and Carsten Flohr.
© 2023 John Wiley & Sons Ltd. Published 2023 by John Wiley & Sons Ltd.
Companion website: www.wiley.com/go/jiyad/handbookofskindiseasemanagement

Dermatitis herpetiformis (DH)

DH is considered a cutaneous manifestation of coeliac disease. Almost all patients will have small bowel findings of gluten-sensitive enteropathy. Ensure they are referred and co-managed with gastroenterology.

All Patients

1) **Skin biopsy for histology (lesional skin) + direct IMF (perilesional skin).**
2) **Serology:** test for tissue transglutaminase (TTG) antibodies (and epidermal transglutaminase if available), endomysial antibodies (EMA), and total IgA (because selective IgA deficiency is relatively common in coeliac disease).
3) **Screen for associated conditions:** thyroid disease (TFTs), diabetes, auto-immune CTDs.

Step 1

All patients generally start with both at outset:
- **Gluten-free diet, GFD** [3]: in a retrospective study where 133 used a GFD, 78% achieved complete control of DH by diet alone. Studies show that a GFD reduces the requirements of dapsone and facilitates discontinuation of this. DH response to diet takes a lot longer than dapsone, months to years.
- **Dapsone** [3]: rapid response to dapsone is a key feature of DH. See page 186 for dosing and monitoring.

Step 2

Where dapsone is contraindicated or not tolerated:
- **Sulfapyridine** [4]: not easily available. Use 500mg TDS, maximum of 6g.
- **Sulfasalazine** [4]: 500mg BD-QDS. Higher doses 1g QDS can be used, as per inflammatory bowel diseases doses.
- **Sulfamethoxypyridine** [3]: not easily available. Use 0.25–1.5g/day.

How accurate are the serological tests for DH?

IgA TTG above 97% specificity, but sensitivity around 50–90%.
IgA EMA testing has specificity close to 100% and sensitivity around 50–100%.
IgA deficiency will reduce test accuracy.

Handbook of Skin Disease Management, First Edition. Zainab Jiyad and Carsten Flohr.
© 2023 John Wiley & Sons Ltd. Published 2023 by John Wiley & Sons Ltd.
Companion website: www.wiley.com/go/jiyad/handbookofskindiseasemanagement

Dermatomyositis (DM)

Dermatomyositis should be managed in conjunction with rheumatologists. Myositis-specific antibodies (**MSAs**) define myositis phenotypes, with each there are specific management requirements (see below). Myositis-associated antibodies (**MAAs**) are not specific to myositis.

All Patients
1) **Full systems review and thorough examination (including malignancy screen).**
2) **Recommend photoprotection.**
3) **Investigations:** FBC, U/E, LFTs, CRP, aldolase, ESR, CK, LDH, MSAs (see below) and MAAs (ANA, Ro/La, dsDNA, anti-Sm, Scl-70, U1RNP, Ku), CXR, ECG, MRI thigh, muscle biopsy, EMG.
4) **Other Ix directed by hx:** PFTs, HRCT, endoscopy, swallow assessment, cardiac enzymes, cardiac MRI, PET-CT/CT, Echo.
5) **Ensure up-to-date malignancy screen.**
6) **Further management is guided by MSA; see below.** If a MSA is not detected or patient considered high risk of malignancy (e.g. tx resistant disease/late onset DM, etc.), perform an extended malignancy screen as outlined below.

DM subtypes
Adult-onset: i) Classic DM, ii) classic DM with malignancy, iii) classic DM part of overlapping CTD, iv) clinically amyopathic DM (CADM), which can be amyopathic or hypomyopathic. **Juvenile-onset (JDM):** i) Classic DM, ii) CADM (amyopathic or hypomyopathic).

Handbook of Skin Disease Management, First Edition. Zainab Jiyad and Carsten Flohr.
© 2023 John Wiley & Sons Ltd. Published 2023 by John Wiley & Sons Ltd.
Companion website: www.wiley.com/go/jiyad/handbookofskindiseasemanagement

MSA	Clinical relevance/phenotype	Specific management
Anti-MDA5	CADM; rapidly progressive interstitial lung disease; cutaneous and oral ulcers; palmar papules; alopecia; panniculitis; arthritis	• PFTS with DLCO: usually repeated at regular intervals for first year (3–4 times). • HRCT. • Refer and co-manage with respiratory team. • Check ferritin – correlates with disease activity. Some advocate testing IL-18 and KL-6 too, if available. • Vasculopathy treatments usually required for ulceration: e.g. nifedipine, sildenafil, pentoxifylline, aspirin, NOACs.
Anti-Mi2	Classic skin signs of DM; mild muscle disease; highly elevated CK; responsive to tx	• Standard treatment approach to DM (overleaf) usually suffices.
Anti-SAE	Severe cutaneous disease but initially relatively mild/absent muscle disease that progresses; associated with dysphagia; fever and weight loss; hydroxychloroquine drug rashes	• Carefully monitor muscle disease (may be misdiagnosed as CADM initially). • Consider avoiding hydroxychloroquine.
Anti-NXP2	Increased risk of malignancy in adults; peripheral oedema; sometimes calcinosis and distal ulcers; severe muscle disease; in children NXP2-JDM associated with significant calcinosis and severe myopathy	• **Extended malignancy screen:** PET-CT or other imaging usually annually, +/- endoscopy, pelvic US, mammogram, further screening as per symptoms. • Calcinosis management outlined below. • Treat NXP2-JDM aggressively.
Anti-TIF1	Strong association with malignancy (20–60%); CADM; severe photosensitive skin disease; palmar hyperkeratosis; ovoid palatal patches, psoriasiform plaques; 'red on white' lesions	• **Extended malignancy screen:** PET-CT or other imaging usually annually, +/- endoscopy, pelvic US, mammogram, further screening as per symptoms.

MSA	Clinical relevance/phenotype	Specific management
Anti-ARS*: **anti-JO-1,** **anti-PL7,** **anti-PL12,** **anti-EJ,** **anti-OJ,** **anti-KS,** **anti-ZO,** **anti-YRS/HA**	Antisynthetase syndrome: ILD, arthritis, fever, Raynaud's, and mechanic's hands	• PFTs with DLCO. • HRCT. • Refer and co-manage with respiratory team.
Anti-SRP*	*Necrotizing myopathy;* severe weakness and very high CK levels	–
Anti-HMGCR*	*Immune-mediated necrotizing myopathy;* increased risk of malignancy; associated with statin use	–
CN1A*	*Inclusion body myositis*	–

*Non-DM-associated MSAs.

Skin only/ CADM

- **TCS** [4]: use BD +/- occlusion. Superpotent for body and moderately potent for face/ neck intertriginous areas.
- **Topical tacrolimus 0.1%** [3]: OD/BD. In a prospective intra-patient study of 5, no significant differences between lesions treated with tacrolimus and untreated lesions. However, there are anecdotal reports of efficacy.
- **Antimalarials** [3]: hydroxychloroquine is antimalarial of choice, 200mg OD/BD (max. 5mg/kg). A retrospective review of patients with CADM found that only 11.4% (10 of 88) treated with hydroxychloroquine achieved adequate response. Quinacrine 100mg OD is usually added in, where hydroxychloroquine monotherapy has failed.
- **Methotrexate** [3]: standard dosing, see page 181. In a retrospective review, 8 of 11 treated with MTX had a significant reduction in both DM skin lesions and CDASI score.
- **If above fail, proceed with MMF > Ciclosporin > IVIG > tofactinib – as below**
- **Adjunctive:** for persistent facial erythema can trial brimonidine gel or clonidine (50 micrograms BD for 2 weeks, increased to 75 micrograms BD); manage pruritus (see page 140).

Systemic disease

- **Systemic steroids** ③: universally initiated, <u>usually 1mg/kg/day; if severe disease/ILD give pulsed methylpred 500mg for 3 consecutive days.</u> Taper dose by ~20–25% monthly. <u>Start concurrent immunosuppressant – below.</u>
- **+/- IVIG** ④: used adjunctively with other immunosuppressants, rapid response. Particularly helpful in cases of infection or malignancy. <u>Dose of 2g/kg.</u> Conflicting evidence, recent placebo-controlled RCT of 26 showed no improvement with IVIG, although previous crossover study of 15 did show an improvement in 70% of patients.

<u>**First-line:**</u> **MTX or azathioprine** ③: <u>standard dosing, see pages 181 and 185.</u> In a retrospective review of 113, MTX and azathioprine were found to be similarly efficacious.

<u>**Second-line:**</u>

- **MMF** ③: preferred starting option for patients with ILD. <u>Standard dosing, see page 188.</u> In a retrospective series of 10 treated with MMF and steroids, 6 were successfully weaned from steroids.
- **Tacrolimus** ③: preferred starting option for patients with ILD. In a retrospective series of 13, 10 improved.
- **Ciclosporin** ③: less commonly used. <u>Standard dosing, see page 183.</u>
- **Combine MTX and azathioprine** ④: of 15 treated with both in a crossover study, 8 improved.

<u>**Third-line – begin with these treatments for severe disease, especially severe ILD:**</u>

- **Rituximab** ④ **OR cyclophosphamide** ③: treatment initiated and managed by rheumatologists.

How to manage calcinosis:

- **Escalate treatment to effectively control DM disease activity.** Some established DM therapies have shown some efficacy for calcinosis: IVIG, rituximab, cyclophosphamide.
- **Diltiazem** ③: *treatment of choice.* Response rates vary from 0 to 64% based on retrospective reviews. Use 60mg BD initially, titrate to maximum dose of 360mg/day.
- **Minocycline** ③: reported response rates 33–88% from small series. Dose: 50–200mg/day (e.g. 50mg BD, 100mg BD).
- **Colchicine** ③: reported response rates of 11–43% from small series. 500 micrograms start at OD and increase to BD after 1 week, as tolerated, to maximum of 2mg.
- **Bisphosphonates** ③: 4 retrospective studies. In 1 retrospective series, of 6 patients treated, 4 had a partial response to alendronate. 10mg daily or 70mg once weekly.
- **Topical or intralesional sodium thiosulphate (STS)** ③: topical STS showed no improvement in 5 DM patients. At least partial response achieved in 5 of 5 calcinosis scleroderma patients with intralesional. IV STS has shown no benefit.
- **Intralesional steroids** ④: case reports from >30 years ago suggest efficacy.
- **Other treatments:** abatacept, infliximab.
- **Interventional options:** can be used adjunctively or principally. Relapse rate is significant. Deep calcinosis is less amenable. Excision, curettage, CO_2 laser, extracorporeal shock-wave therapy, low-frequency ultrasound.

Clinical Pearls

- The risk of malignancy is highest in first year before and after DM diagnosis. The evidence suggests that after 5 years, patients revert to background general population risk. Juvenile DM does not carry a risk of malignancy.
- Consensus treatment algorithms exist for juvenile DM – see Bibliography (online).
- Muscle enzymes can be normal and myositis antibodies are often negative – do not exclude DM diagnosis on the basis of normal CK/other muscle enzymes.
- Several case series have shown good response to tofacitinib for severe refractory cutaneous DM. Benefit may be derived from using this after failure of standard systemics and IVIG, before rituximab.

Dissecting cellulitis of the scalp

As with all scarring alopecias, explain that the **aim** is to treat active disease to prevent further hair loss and that scarred, 'burnt out', areas will not be reversible. As this is scarring, treatment should be escalated appropriately to achieve rapid control.

Active disease is suggested by:

- Symptoms (pain, pruritus, burning, etc.).
- Signs (pustules, nodules, tenderness).
- Ongoing hair loss.
- Active disease on biopsy.

All Patients

1) Take **baseline photographs.**
2) Recommend **hair camouflage** (see Appendix D)/wigs.
3) **Incision and drainage** is widely used to relieve acute symptoms.

At any stage consider tapering course of **oral steroids** (0.5 – 1mg/kg) to stabilise active disease.

> Step 1

- **Tetracyclines** [2]: initiate all patients on a tetracycline, e.g. lymecycline 408mg OD/BD or doxycycline 100mg OD/BD. Treat for 3 months, then taper gradually. In a retrospective study, 4 out of 5 patients had a 'great' reduction in activity.
- **IL corticosteroid injections** [4]: 10mg/mL (5mg/mL for frontal scalp), to particularly active areas.
- **Topical antibiotic/antimicrobial cleanser** [4]: best used *adjunctively*.

Handbook of Skin Disease Management, First Edition. Zainab Jiyad and Carsten Flohr.
© 2023 John Wiley & Sons Ltd. Published 2023 by John Wiley & Sons Ltd.
Companion website: www.wiley.com/go/jiyad/handbookofskindiseasemanagement

Step 2

- **Rifampicin and clindamycin** [4]: <u>BOTH 300mg BD for 10 weeks.</u>
- **Alternative antibiotics** [2]: <u>azithromycin 500mg 3 times weekly for 3 months</u> or <u>ciprofloxacin 500mg BD.</u> In a retrospective review, 3 patients treated with azithromycin showed significant improvement.

Step 3

- **Isotretinoin** [2]: <u>0.5–1mg/kg, review at 3 months.</u> In a retrospective study, 33 of 35 patients experienced complete remission after 3 months. Some recommend this as step 2.

Refractory

- **Dapsone** [4]: <u>see page 186 for dosing.</u>
- **Others:** oral zinc sulphate, TNF α-inhibitors, for localized disease: CO_2 laser, PDT, laser-assisted epilation, surgical excision.

Drug reactions

The key is to distinguish uncomplicated exanthematous (maculopapular) drug reactions from severe cutaneous adverse reactions (SCARs). The table below outlines central distinctive features (in terms of frequency of association) and serves as a **checklist**. These should be assessed with any drug rash consultation. Identification of the culprit agent depends on a thorough drug timeline and knowledge of common culprit agents – *listed overleaf.*

Feature	Exanthematous drug rash	DRESS	AGEP	SJS/TEN
Time-frame	4–21 days	2–6 weeks	24–48 hours	1–3 weeks
Fever	⊖	⊕⊕⊕	⊕⊕⊕	⊕⊕⊕
Lymphadenopathy	⊖	⊕⊕⊕	⊕	⊖
Purpuric/dusky areas (other than legs)	⊖	⊕	⊖	⊕⊕⊕
Blistering	⊖	⊕	⊕	⊕⊕⊕
Epidermal detachment	⊖	⊖	⊖	⊕⊕⊕
Mouth involvement	⊖	⊕⊕	⊕	⊕⊕⊕
Eye involvement	⊖	⊕	⊕	⊕⊕⊕
Targetoid areas	⊕	⊕⊕	⊕	⊕⊕⊕
Facial oedema	⊖	⊕⊕⊕	⊕	⊕
Pustules	⊖	⊕	⊕⊕⊕	⊕
Eosinophilia	⊕⊕	⊕⊕⊕	⊕⊕	⊖
Marked LFT abnormalities	⊖	⊕⊕⊕	⊕	⊕
Renal abnormalities	⊖	⊕⊕	⊕	⊕⊕
Haemodynamically unstable	⊖	⊕⊕	⊕	⊕⊕⊕

Handbook of Skin Disease Management, First Edition. Zainab Jiyad and Carsten Flohr.
© 2023 John Wiley & Sons Ltd. Published 2023 by John Wiley & Sons Ltd.
Companion website: www.wiley.com/go/jiyad/handbookofskindiseasemanagement

Top 10 drug causes for SCARs

DRESS	AGEP	SJS/TEN
Carbamazapine	Penicillins	Allopurinol
Allopurinol	Cephalosporins	Carbamazepine
Phenytoin	Pristinamycin/macrolides	Phenytoin
Lamotrigine	Quinolones	Lamotrigine
Phenobarbital	Hydroxychloroquine	Phenobarbital
Sulfasalazine	Sulphonamides	Co-trimoxazole
Dapsone	Terbinafine	Nevirapine
Vancomycin	Diltiazem	Oxicam NSAIDs
Minocycline	Corticosteroids	Penicillins
Anti-TB drugs	Oxicam NSAIDs	Cephalosporins

SCORTEN and associated mortality

Prognostic factors	Points	SCORTEN	Mortality (%)
Age >40	1	0–1	3
Tachycardia >120 bpm	1	2	12
Malignancy	1	3	35
Initial BSA detached >10%	1	4	58
Serum urea >10 mmol/L	1	5	90
Serum bicarbonate <20 mmol/L	1		
Blood glucose >14 mmol/L	1		

RegiSCAR scoring system for DRESS

Criteria – 1 point for each
Fever $\geq$38.5°C*
Lymphadenopathy ($\geq$1cm and 2 different areas)
Eosinophilia: $\geq$0.7 × 10^9 or $\geq$10% if WBC <4.0 × 10^9 Give *2 points* when $\geq$1.5 × 10^9 or $\geq$20% if WBC <4.0 × 10^9
Atypical lymphocytes on blood film
Rash >50% BSA
Rash suggestive of DRESS*: 2 or more of • purpuric lesions (other than legs). • infiltration. • facial oedema. • psoriasiform desquamation.
Skin biopsy suggesting DRESS*
Organ involvement: score 1 for each organ involved, with a maximum score of 2
Rash resolution $\geq$15 days*
Excluding other causes – score 1 if 3 of the following tests were performed and were all negative: • HAV. • HBV. • HCV. • Mycoplasma. • Chlamydia. • ANA. • Blood culture.

*-1 point if criteria not met.
Total score: <2 = excluded; 2–3 = possible; 4–5 = probable; >6 = definite.

Biopsy all drug rashes? All suspected SCARs should be biopsied, and IMF is usually performed for blistering eruptions for completeness. However, a skin biopsy is not necessary for all uncomplicated exanthematous drug rashes where there is no uncertainty about the diagnosis.

Exanthematous drug rash

- **Treating through is an option if deemed clinically important to continue.**
- **Potent TCS** [4]: provide symptomatic relief.
- **Emollients** [4]: particularly in exfoliative stage.

DRESS

Investigations: FBC, LFTs, renal profile, lipase, blood film, troponin, HHV 6/7, EBV, CMV, ECG, RegiSCAR recommended bloods (hep A,B,C; mycoplasma; chlamydia; ANA; blood culture), CXR.

- **Perform a thorough hx and examination screening for organ involvement.**
- **Immediate withdrawal of causative agent and supportive measures** [4].
- **Potent TCS** [4]: for symptomatic relief.
- **If systemic involvement (e.g. liver, kidney, lung)** [3]: though evidence to suggest benefit is lacking, patients are usually given oral prednisolone at a dose of 0.5–1mg/kg, usually gradually tapered to prevent relapse. Alternatively, pulsed methylprednisolone at a dose of 30mg/kg IV for 3 days. Early initiation is recommended.
- **Ciclosporin** [3]: in a retrospective study, 5 patients treated with ciclosporin had more rapid resolution of fever and lab abnormalities and shorter hospital stay compared with 21 treated with steroids. 3–5mg/kg/day.
- **IVIG NOT recommended** [3]: reports of detrimental effects in some patients (resulting in an open trial being aborted) have dissuaded its use at present.

AGEP

Usually self-resolving in overwhelming majority of patients. Check routine bloods (FBC, renal, and liver).

- **Withdrawal of culprit drug** [4].
- **Potent TCS** [4]: for symptomatic relief.
- **Systemic corticosteroids** [3]: as above for DRESS, can be used in exceptional circumstances where there is systemic involvement.

SJS/TEN

- **Immediate withdrawal of culprit agent** ③: early withdrawal has been shown to reduce mortality considerably in drugs of short half-life (by 30% each day) in an observational study of 203.
- **Admission to ICU/burns unit** ③: prompt discussion with ICU/burns unit should be undertaken for all patients. In a retrospective review, patients treated in a high-care setting had significantly lower mortality.
- **Skin care** ④: nurse on non-adherent sheets (e.g. Exu-Dry®); cover denuded areas with non-adherent dressings (e.g. Mepitel®); deflate but do not deroof blisters; consider use of bear-hugger for thermoregulation; regular 1–2 hourly application of thick emollient (e.g. 50:50 white soft paraffin); consider fecal management system; wash with antibacterial lotion or diluted chlorhexidine.
- **Mucosal surfaces** ④: *mouth* – liberal application of emollient to lips 1–2 hourly. Daily cleansing with sponge/mouthwash. Consider anti-inflammatory oral rinse and steroid mouthwash.

Eyes – early involvement ophthalmology. Regular 2 hourly ocular lubricant. Consider topical antibiotics.

Genito-urinary – daily examination of area. Regular application emollient. Potent TCS to affected, non-denuded areas.

- **Fluid resuscitation and nutritional support:** initial fluid requirements within 24 hours – 2ml/kg/BSA (%) involved; subsequent fluid requirements are to be tailored according to urine output (aiming to achieve 0.5–1ml/kg/hour).
- **Infection surveillance** ④: Regular sampling of blood, skin surfaces, urine. Prophylactic antibiotics not recommended. Antibiotics to be initiated when infection is suspected/positive cultures.
- **Regular systems review and support** ④: e.g. lung, renal, liver, fluid balance. Usually managed by ICU.
- **Pain control** ④: can be severe, consult with pain team/anaesthetics.

Role of immunomodulatory agents remains uncertain. Agents used include the following:

- **Systemic corticosteroids** ③: though evidence from 2 meta-analyses is conflicting, most experts would recommend this first-line, particularly in UK/Europe. Give oral prednisolone or IV methylprednisolone at a dose of 1–2mg/kg; or pulsed methylprednisolone typically at a dose of 250/500/1000mg IV for 3 consecutive days.
- **Ciclosporin** ③: the evidence is favorable. A meta-analysis of 358 found a significant reduction in mortality. Give at a dose of 3–5mg/kg/day. Caution – renal impairment (this selection criteria may have biased studies).
- **TNF inhibitors** ④: RCT of etanercept 25mg or 50mg SC twice weekly vs corticosteroids showed a significant reduction in SCORTEN predicted mortality with etanercept.
- **IVIG** ③: overall, the evidence suggests no real benefit with IVIG. However, some authors believe there is a role for high-dose IVIG (>2mg/kg), although drug complications increase with higher dose.

Should I do any further testing? The diagnosis of drug rashes, including SCARs, is a clinical one. Patch testing, prick testing, and intradermal testing can be useful for determining the culprit drug (when unclear), but otherwise they have little use as diagnostic tests and are not performed in the acute setting.

	Patch testing	Prick testing	Intradermal testing	In vitro testing
Exanthematous (maculopapular)	Can be useful, positive in 10–40%	Unlikely useful	Delayed reading at 24 hours may be useful	Unknown
DRESS	Useful (positive in 32–64%) dependent on drug. Six months after disappearance of rash and other sequelae	Described delayed positive at 24 hours but unknown utility	Delayed reading at 24 hours. Currently unknown safety	For the lymphocyte transformation test (LTT): sensitivity reported 73% and specificity 82%
AGEP	Useful – sensitivity depends on the specific implicated drug (up to 58%)	Unknown	Potentially useful	Unknown
SJS/TEN	Low sensitivity (<30%). Can be considered if there is benefit of diagnostic information obtained	Considered contraindicated	Considered contraindicated	LTT: sensitivity 37%, specificity 98%

What follow-up is needed?

AGEP: usually no long-term sequelae.

DRESS: Several studies have shown the development of autoimmune diseases following DRESS (thyroid, diabetes, vitiligo, alopecia areata). Most experts recommend checking TFTs at 6 months.

SJS/TEN: Ophthalmological sequelae are very common, and patients should be followed up by ophthalmology. Other long-term problems include urinary/vulvovaginal, oral, psychologic, and pulmonary – refer to specialists as appropriate. Cutaneous complications include dyspigmentation (may benefit from camouflage clinic) and pruritus.

Erosive pustular dermatosis of the scalp (EPDS)

EPDS is probably an under-diagnosed condition. Consider in patients with localized areas of pustules, lakes of pus, or crusts overlying eroded nodules/plaques, usually on the balding and UV-damaged scalp of older individuals but also forehead, temples, and lower legs when biopsy has excluded malignancy. EPD can result in scarring and alopecia, and recurrence is common. Evidence for optimal treatment is limited based on SR of heterogeneous case reports and case series.

All Patients

1) Take a **history screening for provoking factors: injuries, burns, topical treatments (e.g. 5-FU), cryotherapy, surgery.**
2) **A biopsy, or multiple biopsies,** should be performed as EPD may simulate malignancy. Histology may be non-specific and many consider EPD to be a diagnosis of exclusion.
3) **Culture** may reveal secondary bacterial infection with staphylococcus aureus; consider fungal scrapes for mycology.

Step 1

- **TCS** [3]: a SR found complete response in 30/80 (38%) patients where TCS monotherapy was used and partial response in 43 (54%) and stable disease in 6/80 (8%). *Trial potent TCS OD for 3–4 weeks.*
- **Topical tacrolimus** [3]: same SR reported complete resolution in 12 of 17 patients (71%) when used as monotherapy. *Use OD for 2–3 months.* Consider introducing with TCS where recurrence or prolonged tx necessary.
- **Topical antibiotic** [3]: same SR reported complete resolution in 4/5 (80%) patients when used as monotherapy (e.g. clindamycin, mupirocin, Fucidin). Usually used in combination with other treatments.

Handbook of Skin Disease Management, First Edition. Zainab Jiyad and Carsten Flohr.
© 2023 John Wiley & Sons Ltd. Published 2023 by John Wiley & Sons Ltd.
Companion website: www.wiley.com/go/jiyad/handbookofskindiseasemanagement

Step 2

- **PDT** ③: in a SR, 14 of 15 had complete resolution. Note, PDT can also be a provoking factor.
- **Oral steroids** ③: in 4 studies of a total of 8 patients, 50% had complete resolution and 38% partial resolution. Use as a weaning regimen, e.g. starting at 25mg OD reducing by 5mg per week. Consider using as combination treatment.

Refractory

- **Oral retinoid** ④: both isotretinoin and acitretin have been used in case reports, with limited success.
- **Others:** topical retinoid, topical calcipotriol, tetracyclines, dapsone, NSAID, Er:YAG laser, oral NSAIDs, oral zinc, methotrexate, tofacitinib.

Erythema multiforme (EM)

EM is considered a distinct entity from SJS/TEN, with drugs being a rare cause of EM. Dividing into minor and major EM (significant mucosal involvement with latter) can help guide treatment. It is important to identify an underlying cause – majority of cases are linked to HSV. History and examination should guide investigations.

Main causes of EM	
Viral	**HSV,** VZV, CMV, EBV, HIV, parapox virus, adenovirus, parvovirus B19, coxsackie, hepatitis
Bacterial	**Mycoplasma pneumoniae,** Chlamydophila psittaci, Mycobacterium tuberculosis, Salmonella
Fungal	Histoplasma capsulatum, dermatophytes
Drugs	NSAIDs, sulphonamides, penicillins, antiepileptics, allopurinol and others
Other	IBD, Behcet's, lupus

EM minor/localised

- **Identify and treat underlying cause.**
- **TCS** ④: potency determined by site.
- **TCS gel/mouthwash for oral involvement** ④: potent/superpotent gels used. If not available, can dissolve betamethasone tablets in water and use as mouthwash (swish and spit), see page 12.
- **Anaesthetic/analgesic/cleansing mouthwash** ④: various preparations available depending on country. See page 12 (aphthous).
- **Refer any ocular involvement to ophthalmologists.**

EM major/widespread

- **Localised therapies as above.**
- **Oral steroids** ③: typically doses of 30–60mg are used. Some dermatologists use a tapering course whilst others use short 5–7-day courses.

Recurrent

- **Aciclovir** ②: 400mg BD for 6 months, then assess. In a placebo-controlled RCT of 20, 7 of 11 patients treated with aciclovir had no attacks during tx.
- **Others:** dapsone, colchicine, levamisole, MMF, azathioprine, thalidomide, hydroxychloroquine, JAK inhibitors.

Handbook of Skin Disease Management, First Edition. Zainab Jiyad and Carsten Flohr.
© 2023 John Wiley & Sons Ltd. Published 2023 by John Wiley & Sons Ltd.
Companion website: www.wiley.com/go/jiyad/handbookofskindiseasemanagement

Erythema nodosum (EN)

History and bloods should screen for secondary causes listed below. Treat the underlying cause, if one is found.

Main causes of EN	
Bacterial	**Streptococcus (most common)**, Mycoplasma pneumonia, Chlamydophila psittaci, Mycobacterium tuberculosis, leprosy, Yersinia, Salmonella
Viral	EBV, hepatitis B, Paravaccinia, HSV, HIV
Fungal	Coccidioidomycosis, histoplasmosis, blastomycosis
Drugs	OCP, penicillins, sulfonamides, bromides and iodides
Other	IBD, lymphoma, leukaemia, solid cancers, sarcoidosis, pregnancy, Whipple's disease, Behcet's, Sweet's, idiopathic

Step 1

- **NSAIDs** [4]: ibuprofen commonly used, although alternatives work as well. 400mg TDS/QDS, can use maximum dose of 2400mg/day.
- **Compression stockings:** useful as adjunctive therapy.

Step 2

- **Oral steroids** [4]: rapidly effective. Typical doses ~30mg for 1 week. If recurrent, consider a slow taper.

Step 3

- **Potassium iodide** [3]: uncommonly used as can be difficult to obtain. In one study, 24 of 28 patients with EN responded to tx. Tablets/granules/drops are diluted to make a saturated solution (SSKI) to be given at a dose of 300mg TDS (consult with pharmacist to do this), usually 2 weeks tx sufficient.

Handbook of Skin Disease Management, First Edition. Zainab Jiyad and Carsten Flohr.
© 2023 John Wiley & Sons Ltd. Published 2023 by John Wiley & Sons Ltd.
Companion website: www.wiley.com/go/jiyad/handbookofskindiseasemanagement

> **Refractory/ recurrent**
>
> All based on case reports/expert opinion.
>
> - **Hydroxychloroquine** [4]: case reports suggest benefit. Typically 200mg BD used.
> - **Colchicine** [4]: 500 micrograms 2–4 times/day (max 6mg). Nausea/diarrhoea usually limit dose titrations.
> - **Dapsone** [4]: see page 186 for dose and monitoring.
> - **Other** [4] : TNF-alpha inhibitors, MMF, tetracycline, erythromycin.

Female pattern hair loss

All Patients

1) **Bloods:** evidence limited but usually recommended that ferritin levels are >70. Some dermatologists recommend checking and correcting B12, folate + TFTs as well. Androgen profile only recommended if there are other signs/symptoms of androgen excess.
2) **Baseline and follow-up standardised, global photography** to assess response.
3) Recommend **hair camouflage** (see Appendix D)/wigs.

Clinical Pearl

Best results are likely achieved by *combining* treatments for particularly motivated patients: e.g. minoxidil + spironolactone.

Step 1

- **Topical minoxidil** [1]: typically 5% is used, though studies have found no significant difference between 2% vs 5%. Foam preparation has no propylene glycol, which can cause irritation. Treat for at least 6–12 months before assessing efficacy. Counsel re: potential transient increase in hair shedding in first 3 months. Hair loss will have progressed on discontinuation, so treatment should continue indefinitely.

Handbook of Skin Disease Management, First Edition. Zainab Jiyad and Carsten Flohr.
© 2023 John Wiley & Sons Ltd. Published 2023 by John Wiley & Sons Ltd.
Companion website: www.wiley.com/go/jiyad/handbookofskindiseasemanagement

Step 2

- **Spirinolactone** ③: in a single open-intervention study of 80 women, half were given spironolactone and half cyproterone acetate; 44% of the *combined group* showed hair regrowth. Start at 25–50mg OD and gradually increase to maximum of 200mg/day, see page 193. Continue for at least 12 months to assess efficacy.
- **Low-dose oral minoxidil (0.25–5mg)** ③: recent observational pilot study of 100 women treated with spironolactone (25mg) and low-dose oral minoxidil (0.25mg) identified a mean reduction in Sinclair hair loss severity scale of 0.85 at 6 and 1.3 at 12 months. A retrospective, multicenter review of 1404 patients (943, 67.2% female) revealed adverse events (in order of frequency: hypertrichosis, lightheadedness, fluid retention, tachycardia, headache, periorbital oedema, and insomnia) in almost 21%, but insufficient to cause treatment discontinuation in 98.3%, and no serious adverse events were recorded.
- **Cyproterone acetate with OCP** ③ (*Dianette®*): Evidence from above study. Thrombosis risk considered high and infrequently prescribed. Dianette is pre-prepared form, otherwise prescribe as 50mg of cyproterone on days 1–10 of menstrual cycle and 35 mcg on ethinyl estradiol on days 1–21 OR 100mg/day on days 5–15 and 50 mcg of ethinyl estradiol on days 5–25. Recent concerns have been raised about the risk of meningioma.

Step 3

- **Low-level laser light therapy (LLLT)** ②: RCT of 42 women LLLT vs sham device found 37% increase in hair growth in the active treatment group as compared to the placebo group. Generally used as *adjunctive* treatment. Patient purchases product for home use and follows instructions of device.
- **Other:** finasteride, bicalutamide, microneedling, mesotherapy, platelet-rich plasma, hair transplant.

Treatment depends on identifying the cause of flushing - most common causes listed on the next page.

Investigations
How to investigate?

History should screen for cause. If unclear/non-physiologic/non-rosacea cause, then key investigations as follows:

- **Carcinoid syndrome:** 24-hr urine collection for 5-HIAA and serum serotonin.
- **Phaeochromocytoma:** 24-hr urine for metanephrines, VMA (vanillylmandelic acid) and NE (norepinephrine) or plasma metanephrines.
- **Mastocytosis:** serum tryptase, serum histamine, and consider 24-hr urine for prostaglandin D2 metabolites.
- **TFTs.**
- **Other investigations** directed by history: VIP level, imaging. etc.

Treatment

- **Discontinue causative medications.**
- **Treat the underlying cause, where possible.**
- **Rosacea:** see page 151.
- **Physiologic:** – *beta-blockers* widely used, e.g. <u>propranolol 40mg OD.</u>
  - *Clonidine*, an α-2 adrenergic agonist, also widely used, <u>50 micrograms BD, increased to 75 micrograms BD as necessary.</u>
  - *SSRIs* such as fluoxetine have shown benefit in improving hot flushes in climacteric flushing, e.g. <u>fluoxetine 20mg OD.</u>
  - *Psychological treatments* can help modify biofeedback in emotional flushing.
  - *Hormone replacement therapy* can improve climacteric flushing.
  - *Sympathectomy* is a last resort, and side effects can be severe.

Handbook of Skin Disease Management, First Edition. Zainab Jiyad and Carsten Flohr.
© 2023 John Wiley & Sons Ltd. Published 2023 by John Wiley & Sons Ltd.
Companion website: www.wiley.com/go/jiyad/handbookofskindiseasemanagement

Causes

Physiologic flushing (common)
- Emotion.
- Thermoregulatory (fever).
- Food or beverage.
- Climacteric (menopause).

Rosacea (common)
Alcohol
Medication
- *Oral:* NSAIDs, opiates, vasodilators, cholinergics, steroids, calcium channel blockers, serotonin agonists, contrast media, catecholamines, vancomycin, rifampicin.
- *Topical:* cinnamic aldehyde, brimonidine.

Food
- Nitrites (deli meats/cured meats).
- Sulfites (common additive/preservative).
- Capsaicin (spicy food).
- Scromboid fish poisoning.

Hyperthyroidism
Carcinoid syndrome
Phaeochromocytoma
Mastocytosis
Infusion reactions/hypersensitivity
Pancreatic cell tumour (VIP tumour)
Renal cell carcinoma
Medullary thyroid carcinoma
Neurological
- Migraine, Parkinson's, Horner syndrome, Frey syndrome, others.

Infectious causes	Non-infectious causes
Bacterial **Staphylococcus** • Topical antibiotics (mupirocin, erythromycin). • Antibacterial wash (e.g. Dermol 500® lotion). • Flucloxacillin if widespread or severe. • If recurrent: eradicate S. aureus carriage (mupirocin applied to nostrils and chlorhexidine wash, both daily for 5 days). • Consider long course of tetracyclines. **Pseudomonas 'hot tub folliculitis'** • Usually self-resolves, but oral ciprofloxacin can be used if severe. **Gram negative folliculitis** • Treat with oral isotretinoin (standard dosing, see page 189).	**Normal flora/culture negative folliculitis** • *Most common cause of folliculitis.* • Avoid sweating. • Avoid shaving against hair direction. • Avoid tight clothing. • Antibacterial lotion as shower gel. • Combined antibacterial/steroid creams can provide some relief. • Consider long course of tetracyclines. • Consider isotretinoin. • Consider laser hair removal.
Fungal **Dermatophytes** • See page 165. Majocchi's granuloma usually requires systemic antifungals. **Candida** • Treat with topical azoles (page 220) or short course of oral fluconazole. **Pityrosporum** • Treat with oral itraconazole 200mg OD for 1–2 weeks. • Recurrence is common; weekly use of antifungal shampoos as shower gel +/- pulsed itraconazole 200mg BD for only 1 day per month.	**Irritation associated** • As above.
Demodex • Topical permethrin/oral metronidazole/oral ivermectin.	**Eosinophilic folliculitis:** treat underlying cause
	Drug-induced: stop drug, see list of causes page 206

Folliculitis decalvans

As with all scarring alopecias, explain that the **aim** is to treat active disease to prevent further hair loss and that scarred; 'burnt out' areas will usually not be reversible.

Active disease is suggested by:

- Symptoms (itching, pain, burning, etc.).
- Inflammation (pustules, erythema, crust).
- Ongoing hair loss.
- Active disease on biopsy.

All Patients

1) Take **baseline photographs.**
2) Recommend **hair camouflage** (see Appendix D)/wigs.
3) Take bacterial and fungal **swabs.**
4) Swab for **nasal Staph. carriage** if recurrent infections.

At any stage consider tapering course of **oral steroids** (0.5–1mg/kg) to stabilise active disease.

Step 1

Best results likely achieved with combination of below:

- **Tetracyclines** [2]: initiate all patients on a tetracycline, e.g. lymecycline 408mg OD or doxycycline 100mg OD. Treat for 3 months, then taper gradually. In a retrospective study, 90% of 39 patients treated with tetracyclines showed some response.
- **Potent/superpotent TCS** [2]: use adjunctively OD to active areas, assess at 3 month and taper gradually, consider in combination with **IL corticosteroid injections** [2] 10mg/mL (5mg/mL for frontal scalp) to particularly active areas.
- **Topical clindamycin** [3]: for mild disease only, combined with TCS. Do not combine with oral antibiotics.

Handbook of Skin Disease Management, First Edition. Zainab Jiyad and Carsten Flohr.
© 2023 John Wiley & Sons Ltd. Published 2023 by John Wiley & Sons Ltd.
Companion website: www.wiley.com/go/jiyad/handbookofskindiseasemanagement

Step 2

- **Rifampicin and clindamycin** ③: <u>BOTH 300mg BD for 10 weeks.</u> A retrospective study showed that all 15 patients treated with this improved, with disease remission at an average of 7.2 months.
- **Azithromycin** ③: alternative if above not tolerated. All three patients treated with this in a retrospective review improved. <u>Prescribe 500mg 3 times weekly for 3 months.</u>

Step 3

- **Isotretinoin** ②: <u>0.1–1mg/kg/day.</u> A retrospective series of 39 patients found that 36 achieved partial or complete success following up to 8 months of tx. Antibacterial co-treatment often used initially to control infection.

Refractory

- **Others:** dapsone ④ <u>(see page 186 for dosing)</u>.
- **Limited evidence:** TNF α-inhibitors, Nd:YAG laser, PDT, Ciclosporin.

Frontal fibrosing alopecia (FFA)

Considered a subtype of **lichen planopilaris**. See LPP on page 95 for signs/symptoms of active disease.

As with all scarring alopecias, explain that the **aim** is to treat active disease to prevent further hair loss and that scarred, 'burnt out' areas will not be reversible.

All Patients

1) **Biopsy:** using scarring alopecia biopsy protocol (page 217).
2) Take **baseline photographs.**
3) Recommend **hair camouflage** (see Appendix D)/wigs.
4) Record **baseline measurements** as follows, to facilitate monitoring:

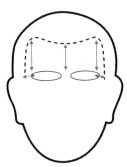

i) Glabella to hairline.
ii) Left outer canthus to hairline.
iii) Right outer canthus to hairline.
iv) Left outer canthus to sideburn.
v) Right outer canthus to sideburn.

At any stage consider tapering course of **oral steroids** (0.5 – 1mg/kg) to stabilise active disease.

Handbook of Skin Disease Management, First Edition. Zainab Jiyad and Carsten Flohr.
© 2023 John Wiley & Sons Ltd. Published 2023 by John Wiley & Sons Ltd.
Companion website: www.wiley.com/go/jiyad/handbookofskindiseasemanagement

Step 1

- **Potent/superpotent TCS** ③: <u>use OD/BD</u> to active areas, sometimes consider with <u>concurrent</u> use of **topical calcineurin inhibitors** ③, if tolerated. Taper TCS when improves. Restart for flares.
- **AND/OR IL corticosteroid injections** ③: <u>(2.5–5mg/mL)</u> to active edge, every 4–6 weeks.
- **Topical minoxidil** ④: <u>Use 5%.</u> Consider a trial of this for at least 4 months to assess efficacy; explain this would only influence undamaged hair follicles. Foam preparation has no propylene glycol, which can cause irritation (especially in inflamed scalp).
- Treat **androgenetic alopecia** if present (see page 57).

Step 2

- **Hydroxychloroquine** ③: all but mild cases should be initiated on <u>200mg BD or OD</u> (max. 5mg/kg). In a retrospective review of published cases, 17 of 23 patients (74%) treated with hydroxychloroquine monotherapy showed improvement.

Step 3

- **5-α reductase inhibitors** ③: in a review of the literature, <u>finasteride (1–5mg/day) or dutasteride (0.5mg/day)</u> were found to stabilise hair loss in 88% of 180 total cases (low-level evidence). Some dermatologists recommend use of these prior to hydroxychloroquine.

Step 4

- **Retinoids** ③: a retrospective review of 54 patients found that treatment with either <u>isotretinoin (20mg OD) or acitretin (20mg OD)</u> for 1 year stabilised hair loss in ~75% of patients.
- **Alternatively, doxycycline** ③: <u>100mg BD</u>, though evidence suggests limited efficacy.

Refractory

- **Methotrexate** ④: see page 181 for initiation, dosing, and management of complications.
- **Others:** MMF, naltrexone, pioglitazone (a retrospective review showed 3 of 4 patients on <u>15mg/day</u> responded to treatment; likely best used as *adjunct* therapy; low-level evidence overall).

Graft-versus-host disease (GVHD)

GVHD is a multisystem disorder, necessitating good multidisciplinary care. Although there is significant overlap between **acute (<100 days) vs chronic GVHD (>100 days)**, the distinction is still used to guide treatment. Management of acute GVHD (aGVHD) is highly dependent on grade, with mortality increasing with increasing grade. A careful balance needs to be struck **between GVHD and graft-versus-tumour effect**, as over-immunosuppression may result in a detrimental effect.

All Patients with any Form of Cutaneous GVHD:

1) **Advise sun protection.**
2) **Regular use of emollients.**
3) **Avoidance of strongly fragranced products.**
4) **Recognise and manage GVHD triggers, where possible:** infections, drug reactions, recent decrease in immunosuppression, break in extracorporeal photophoresis (ECP), donor lymphocyte infusions (DLI).

Grading of acute GVHD (Glucksberg)

		Extent of organ involvement		
		Skin	Liver	Gut
Stage	**1**	<25% of skin affected	Bilirubin 2-3mg/dl	Diarrhoea >500ml/day or persistent nausea
	2	25-50% of skin affected	Bilirubin 3-6mg/dl	Diarrhoea >1000ml/day
	3	>50% of skin affected	Bilirubin 6-15mg/dl	Diarrhoea >1500ml/day
	4	Erythroderma with bullae	Bilirubin >15mg/dl	Severe abdominal pain with or without ileus
Grade	**I**	Stage 1-2	None	None
	II	Stage 3	Stage 1	Stage 1
	III	Stage 1-3	Stage 2-3	Stage 2-4
	IV	Stage 4	Stage 4	-

Source: Adapted from Glucksberg H, Storb R, Fefer A, et al. Clinical manifestations of graft-versus-host disease in human recipients of marrow from hl-a-matched sibling donors1. Transplantation [Internet] 1974 [cited 2021 May 31];18(4):295–304. Available from: https://pubmed.ncbi.nlm.nih.gov/4153799/.

Management of <u>acute</u> GVHD:

Grade 1 disease

- **Topical corticosteroids** ④: variable potency used depending on site, <u>OD/BD.</u>
- **Optimise levels of oral calcineurin inhibitors** ④: these are usually given by haematologists to most patients as prophylaxis for GVHD, and the dose can be optimised to control GVHD. *For those who are not on calcineurin inhibitors,* usually these are initiated first-line alongside steroids, as below.

Grade 2 disease

- **As per grade 1. Consult and co-manage with haematologists.**
- **Initiate methylprednisolone at dose of 1mg/kg/day** ②.

Grade 3–4 disease

- **As per grade 1. Consult and co-manage with haematologists.**
- **Initiate methylprednisolone at dose of 2mg/kg/day** ③.

When systemic steroids fail

No consensus to support one particular treatment of below. The choice of treatment will depend on organ involvement and centre preference and will be guided by haematologists:

- **MMF** ③: one study found skin responded better to MMF than other organs involved.
- **Extracorporeal photophoresis (ECP)** ②: in a randomised phase II study, steroids + ECP was found to be superior to steroids alone for the treatment of grade II–IV aGVHD. Further, ECP was more effective in treating skin GVHD, compared with other organs.
- **Ruxolitinib** ②: in phase III study of ruxolitinib vs other standard treatments, ruxolitinib performed better.
- **mTOR inhibitors** ③: uncontrolled studies report response rates just over 50%.
- **IL-2 antibodies** ③: an uncontrolled study of 64 patients reported a total response rate of 84% with daclizumab.
- **Anti-TNF drugs** ③: mainly used where there is marked GI involvement.

Refractory

Choice of treatment guided by haematologists: alemtuzumab (Campath®), antithymocyte globulin, pentostatin, mesenchymal stem cells, methotrexate.

Management of <u>chronic</u> GVHD:

> The National Institutes of Health (NIH) GHVD scoring system is used to grade chronic GVHD. An app is available to facilitate scoring: 'eGVHD'. Grade/severity generally dictates initiating treatment, as per options below.

Step 1

- **Topical corticosteroids** [4]: variable potency used depending on site, <u>OD/BD.</u>
- **Topical calcineurin inhibitors** [4]: uncommonly used, <u>OD/BD.</u>

Step 2

- **Continue topicals as above.** [3]
- **Initiate prednisolone at dose of 1mg/kg/day:** taper the dose slowly.
- **Oral calcineurin inhibitors** [3]: tacrolimus or ciclosporin initiated/dose optimised. Often this is done when systemic steroids are initiated.

Step 3

- **ECP** [2]: high response rates reported with cutaneous chronic GVHD.
- **Consider with haematology discussion:** pentostatin, rituximab, or imatinib (for sclerodermatous GVHD).

Refractory

No consensus/strong evidence to support one particular treatment of below:
- **PUVA phototherapy** [3]: is an option where skin is particularly resistant. One study reported 37% achieved complete remission.
- **MMF, methotrexate, or pulse steroids** [3]: frequently used.
- **Other treatments initiated by haematologists, depend on local centre preference:** ibrutinib, JAK inhibitors, mTOR inhibitors, proteosome inhibitors.

Oral GVHD – in addition to above, certain other measures may be useful:

- **Potent topical corticosteroids:** in oral-friendly form, see page 12.
- **Topical tacrolimus.**
- **Antimicrobial and anti-inflammatory agents:** e.g. chlorhexidine, doxycycline, and nystatin mouthwashes, see page 12.
- **Analgesia:** e.g. lidocaine spray, see page 12.
- **Oral lubricants and salivary stimulants.**

Granuloma annulare (GA)

The evidence for associations with various conditions, including diabetes, malignancy, and hyperlipidaemia, is inconclusive. In general, screening tests are *not* necessary when a diagnosis of GA is made. Tx is largely dictated by two factors: **i) subtype** (localised, generalised, subcutaneous, perforating, patch, etc.), which determines likely chronicity (generalised is more likely to be chronic/ relapsing-remitting), and **ii) presence/absence of symptoms,** e.g. tenderness (subcutaneous GA) or itchiness (generalised GA). The condition is generally self-limiting, and tx is not always indicated.

Step 1

Best for localised GA:

- **Potent/superpotent TCS** [4]: use OD or BD. Need to trial for 4–6 weeks before evaluating efficacy. Consider under occlusion. Slowly taper if improving.
- **Intralesional steroids** [3]: 10mg/mL injections can be used to localised, resistant areas. Warn re: risk of atrophy.
- **Topical tacrolimus** [4]: less commonly used. Case series of 4, 2 improved with BD use of tacrolimus 0.1%.

Step 2

Consider these first-line for generalised GA:

- **Phototherapy** [3]: more evidence exists for PUVA than NBUVB, but both with studies showing complete/partial remission in over half of patients with generalised GA.
- **Hydroxychloroquine** [3]: 200mg OD or BD. In a retrospective study of 35 patients with generalised/subcutaneous GA, 55% of those treated with hydroxychloroquine improved. 100% of chloroquine-treated patients improved.

Granuloma annulare (GA)

Refractory

- **Methotrexate** ③: in a retrospective review of 11, 64% improved, of which 43% showing complete clearance. Mean tx duration was 11 months.
- **Isotretinoin** ④: case reports have shown improvement/remission with doses of ~0.5–1mg/kg/day.
- **Dapsone** ③: in an uncontrolled study of 10, 7 responded to tx with dapsone.
- **Biologics** ③: best evidence for adalimumab (study of 7). There are case reports of infliximab success.
- **Fumaric acid esters** ②: retrospective study of 8, all showed some improvement except 1, but 6 had side effects.
- **Others** ④: ciclosporin, oral steroids (usually relapse), tofacitinib, aprelimast, doxycycline, pentoxifylline, colchicine, hydroxyurea, nicotinamide, rifampicin + oxofloxacin + minocycline, laser, cryotherapy, imiquimod, PDT.

G

Grover's disease

Often no treatment is necessary, unless symptomatic or appearance troubles the patient. Though some cases are persistent, often it runs an intermittent course. A SR reported time course to spontaneous resolution ranging from 1 week to 8 months.

Encourage All Patients to Avoid Recognised Triggers

- Excessive sweating.
- Sunlight.
- Tight clothing/occlusion.
- Ionising radiation.

Step 1

- **Topical corticosteroids** [3]: used first-line, variable potency used. OD/BD. A SR reported complete response in 31 of 44 patients treated with TCS (70%).
- **Topical calcineurin inhibitors** [3]: some case reports of success. Use OD/BD.
- **Other topicals** [3]: retinoids, antibiotics.

Step 2

- **Oral retinoids** [3]: an SR reported 30 of 35 (86%) of patients improved. See page 189 for initiation, use low-dose isotretinoin or acitretin.

Refractory

- **Oral steroids** [3]: a short course of systemic steroids can be useful in resistant cases.
- **Tetracyclines** [3]: a case series reported 2 out 5 patients improved with tetracycline.
- **PUVA** [4]: case reports of improvement.
- **Others:** dapsone, ciclosporin, etanercept.

Handbook of Skin Disease Management, First Edition. Zainab Jiyad and Carsten Flohr.
© 2023 John Wiley & Sons Ltd. Published 2023 by John Wiley & Sons Ltd.
Companion website: www.wiley.com/go/jiyad/handbookofskindiseasemanagement

Hailey-Hailey disease

The evidence for treatment of Hailey-Hailey disease is very limited and largely based on case reports and case series.

All Patients

1) A **biopsy with immunofluorescence** is necessary to distinguish Hailey-Hailey from other acantholytic disorders.
2) Recommend **chlorhexidine wash.**
3) **Keep skin cool, avoid friction, and use absorbent pads, advise weight loss if appropriate.**

Clinical Pearl

If poorly responsive to treatment or any clinical suspicion, swab for HSV and treat with acyclovir, as appropriate.

Step 1

- **Moderately potent–potent TCS** [3]: use OD/BD. Intermittent use. In a cross-sectional study of 58, 86% found TCS helpful.
- **Topical antifungals** [4]: clotrimazole 1% or econazole 1% use OD/BD.
- **Topical tacrolimus 0.1%** [4]: use OD/BD. Evidence from case reports and case series.
- **Topical antibiotics** [3]: clindamycin/mupirocin/gentamicin creams most frequently used.

Step 2

- **Botulinum toxin (Botox) injections** [4]: case series/reports of injections to axillary area show benefit.
- **Oral erythromycin/tetracyclines** [3]: erythromycin 500mg BD or doxycycline 100mg OD/BD. In a review of 58 patients, 25 (48%) improved with oral erythromycin or penicillin.
- **Naltrexone** [4]: case series show improvement with doses of 1.5–3mg once nightly, can be titrated to 4.5mg.

Refractory

- **Retinoids** [4]: acitretin 10–25mg OD, or alitretinoin 20–30mg OD.
- **Methotrexate** [4]: see page 181 for dosing.
- **Ciclosporin** [4]: see page 183 for dosing.
- **Interventional** [4]: excision, laser, PDT, dermabrasion.
- **Others** [4]: oral magnesium chloride, oral steroids (for severe flares), oral glycopyrrolate, topical 5-FU, topical calcipotriol, thalidomide, dapsone, etanercept, apremilast, UVB.

Hidradenitis suppurativa (HS)

Staging, using the Hurley staging system, is useful to prognosticate and to guide treatment. Objective scoring measures such as HiSCR and HS PGA are useful for monitoring progress and response to treatment. **Severity of disease** determines treatment stage and therapy, e.g. in some patients, rifampicin and clindamycin may be the initiating treatment. Patients may benefit from an **MDT** approach (plastic surgery, microbiology, and psychology).

All Patients

1) **Take a history screening for comorbidities:** cardiovascular disease, PCOS, depression, diabetes, malignancies, acne, IBD. Enquire about family history of HS.
2) **Bloods:** consider bloods for diabetes and hyperlipidaemia.
3) **Encourage weight loss and smoking cessation.**
4) **Consider analgesics for pain management.**

The pathogenesis of HS is thought to be *multifactorial*, hence, a *multifaceted* approach to treatment, illustrated the diagram below, is recommended. *Acute/ interventional* tx can be employed at any point and interweaves medical therapies: it is suggested that medical therapy, including biologics, does not need to be discontinued perioperatively and that continuation may actually result in better outcomes. Escalation of therapy does not necessarily mean cessation of previous tx, and it is believed that better results are achieved by **combining** therapies. Case examples:

MILD: topicals + oral tetracycline.
MODERATE: topicals + oral tetracycline + OCP.
SEVERE: topicals + acitretin + metformin + OCP + adalimumab.

Additionally, try to factor in comorbidities when considering tx options:

- Metformin if there is concurrent diabetes/PCOS.
- Retinoid if patient also has acne.
- Spironolactone if evidence of androgenetic alopecia.

Handbook of Skin Disease Management, First Edition. Zainab Jiyad and Carsten Flohr.
© 2023 John Wiley & Sons Ltd. Published 2023 by John Wiley & Sons Ltd.
Companion website: www.wiley.com/go/jiyad/handbookofskindiseasemanagement

Hidradenitis suppurativa (HS)

H

Interventional/Acute – Consider these Treatments for Flares at Any Stage, Where Appropriate:

- **IL triamcinolone** ③: use 10mg/mL injected directly into acute lesions.
- **Prednisolone** ④: 0.5–1mg/kg. Can use short (1-week courses), longer weaning course (typically 6 weeks), or pulsed doses.
- **Deroofing/punch debridement** ②: though incision and drainage has traditionally been used, this has a high recurrence rate, and punch debridement/deroofing is widely accepted as a superior technique.
- **Wide local excision/CO₂ laser:** consider for severe disease or localised/recurrent.
- **Ertapenem** ③: 1g/daily for 6 weeks intravenously. Reserve as rescue therapy for severe flare (pre-biologic) or pre-surgery. A retrospective review of 30 patients found that 67% (29/43) and 26% (13/50) of Hurley stage 1 and 2 areas reached clinical remission after ertapenem, respectively.

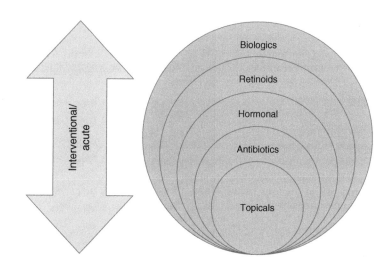

Step 1

All patients are initiated on topicals in conjunction with tetracycline antibiotics, unless very mild disease, in which case topicals alone may be trialled.

TOPICALS:

- **Cleanser** ④: chlorhexidine, Octenisan (best tolerated), zinc pyrithione, or benzoyl peroxide. Start at twice/week during showering and increase up as tolerated. No evidence exists to suggest one is superior to the other.
- **Resorcinol 15%** ②: an antiseptic and keratolytic applied directly to active lesions BD. Caution – can cause contact dermatitis. Not used in UK.
- **Topical clindamycin 1% solution** ④: use BD. A 12-week placebo-controlled RCT of 27 found reduction in number of pustules, when compared to placebo.

TETRACYCLINE ANTIBIOTICS ④:

- doxycycline 100mg BD/tetracycline 500mg BD/lymecycline 408mg OD/minocycline 100mg OD/BD (evidence for minocycline less robust). Use for at least 3–4 months continuously to assess efficacy. 16-week RCT comparing tetracycline vs clindamycin solution found 30% reduction of abscesses in both groups, with no significant difference between the 2 groups.

- **Topical retinoids** ④: may be of benefit with comedonal subtype.

Step 2

- **Rifampicin and clindamycin** ②: BOTH 300mg BD for 10–12 weeks. A SR reported response rates of 71–93% in 187 patients. Courses can be repeated intermittently.

Step 3

Alternative Antibiotics:

- **Rifampicin (300mg BD) + moxifloxacin (400mg OD) + metronidazole (500mg TDS)** ②: in a retrospective review, 8 of 10 with Hurley stage II and 2 of 12 patients with Hurley stage III had complete response.
- **Dapsone** ②: in a retrospective review of 24, only 25% (6 patients) achieved significant improvement.

AND/OR Hormonal:

- **Metformin** ③: start at 500mg OD and increase to BD/TDS. 18 of 25 patients improved in a 24-week prospective trial. Consider especially in PCOS/diabetes.
- **Cyproterone acetate** ④: 1 RCT compared with ethinyl estradiol/noregestrol and improvement found with both groups, with no significant difference. See page 58 for dosing.
- **Spironolactone** ③: in a retrospective review of 20, 85% reported improvement, with complete remission in 55%. Consider especially if concurrent androgenetic alopecia. See page 193 for dosing.
- **Finasteride** ④: case reports with doses ranging from 1.25 to 5mg/day have reported some success.

AND/OR Retinoids:

- **Acitretin** ③: though evidence not robust, this is considered to be superior to isotretinoin. In a prospective study of 17, approximately half improved. <u>Start at 25mg/day and increase gradually.</u>
- **Isotretinoin** ③: best for patients with concurrent acne. Overall, data from uncontrolled studies showed that 85 of 207 (41%) improved. <u>Start at 20mg OD and increase as required.</u>

Step 4

- **Adalimumab** ④: <u>initiate at 160mg SC (single dose or split 80-mg doses given over 2 consecutive days), then 80mg on day 15, then 40mg once weekly starting on day 29.</u> In PIONEER I study, 42% vs 26% (placebo) improved. Above txs may need to be continued alongside biologics.
- **Infliximab** ④: <u>use 5mg/kg every 8 weeks.</u> If adalimumab fails, this can be trialled as alternative. Four-weekly doses have been suggested if patients flare between doses.

Other

- **Limited evidence for efficacy** ②: ciclosporin.
- **Emerging/anecdotal:** secukinumab, golimumab, anakinra, ustekinumab, zinc gluconate (90mg/day).
- **Not recommended:** azathioprine, methotrexate and etanercept.

Hirsutism

Investigating hirsutism depends on the history and menopausal state (pre/post). The Ferriman-Gallwey score is useful for assessing severity and response to treatment (see next page). Causes of hirsutism are outlined overleaf. This treatment algorithm largely pertains to hirsutism secondary to PCOS and idiopathic hirsutism (the underlying causes in the majority of cases).

All Patients

1) **Detailed history:** timing, medication history, virilisation, PCOS/other medical problems.
2) **Bloods:** check serum testosterone and SHBG to give a free androgen index – see overleaf for investigations algorithm.

Step 1

- **Combined oral contraceptive pill** ③: opt for a COC with nonadrogenic progestins (e.g. Yasmin®) or containing an antiandrogen such as cyproterone acetate (e.g. Dianette®, see page 58). Caution VTE risk.
- **Hair reduction methods** ③: long-lasting effects can be achieved with electrolysis and lasers.
- **Eflornithine cream** ④: generally no longer used as monotherapy, but some evidence for improved outcomes when combined with laser hair removal.

Step 2

- **Spironolactone** ①: *antiandrogen of choice.* A Cochrane review showed a subjective but not objective improvement in hirsutism, although a different meta-analysis did show reduction in Ferriman-Gallwey score. See Appendix A for dosing.
- **Finasteride** ①: 2.5–5mg/day. Meta-analysis found no significant differences between spironolactone and finasteride.
- **Flutamide NOT RECOMMENDED:** although effective for hirsutism, there are strong concerns regarding hepatoxicity.

Clinical pearl: COC should be combined with antiandrogen in most cases to prevent pregnancy, and it is likely that this pairing enhances treatment results.

Handbook of Skin Disease Management, First Edition. Zainab Jiyad and Carsten Flohr.
© 2023 John Wiley & Sons Ltd. Published 2023 by John Wiley & Sons Ltd.
Companion website: www.wiley.com/go/jiyad/handbookofskindiseasemanagement

Metformin: a SR and meta-analysis of RCTs found no significant reduction in hirsutism based on Ferriman-Gallwey criteria. Hence, it is not recommended for the treatment of hirsutism.

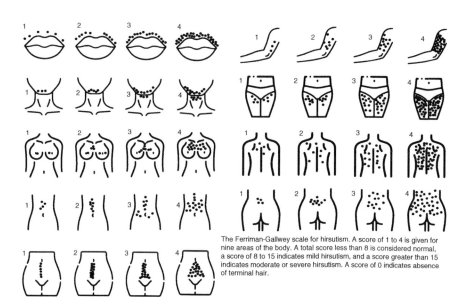

The Ferriman-Gallwey scale for hirsutism. A score of 1 to 4 is given for nine areas of the body. A total score less than 8 is considered normal, a score of 8 to 15 indicates mild hirsutism, and a score greater than 15 indicates moderate or severe hirsutism. A score of 0 indicates absence of terminal hair.

Source: Modified from Somani N, Harrison S, Bergfeld WF. The clinical evaluation of hirsutism. Dermatol Ther 2008;21(5):376–91.

Causes

Ovarian
- Polycystic ovary syndrome.
- Insulin-resistance syndromes.
- Hyperandrogenism, insulin resistance, acanthosis nigricans (HAIR-AN).
- Hyperthecosis.
- Familial ovarian hyperplasia.
- Hilus cell hyperplasia.
- Ovarian tumours.

Adrenal
- Classical congenital adrenal hyperplasia (CAH).
- Nonclassical (late-onset) CAH.
- Cushing's syndrome.
- Adrenal virilising tumours.

Pituitary
- Cushing's disease.
- Acromegaly.
- Hyperprolactinemia.

Idiopathic
- Occult functional hyperandrogenism.
- Increased peripheral 5α-reductase activity.
- Altered androgen receptor function.

Pregnancy
- Aromatase deficiency in the fetus.
- Luteoma of pregnancy.
- Hyperreactio luteinalis.

Exogenous
- Androgenic medications

If moderate hirsutism (F-G score >15) or any suggestion of hyperandrogenism: plasma total or free testosterone level and SHBG. *this can be falsely low if on OCP*	Testosterone level normal: No further testing usually required.	Further testing: Dehydroepiandrosterone sulfate (DHEAS)
	Testosterone level 2.4–7 nmol/L (70–200 ng/dL): Early morning plasma levels of total and free and testosterone. If free levels are high – proceed as below.	Androstenedione Dihydrotestosterone Follicle-stimulating hormone (FSH) Luteinising hormone (LH) Serum oestradiol Serum prolactin 17-hydroxyprogesterone (for CAH) TFTs
	Testosterone level >7 nmol/L (>200 ng/dL): urgent US/CT, further testing as outlined, and refer to endocrinology	

Figure: how to investigate hirsutism. Society guidelines and expert opinions advise no investigations for mild hirsutism without features of hyperandrogenism.

PCOS diagnostic criteria

Two of three criteria must be fulfilled, in adolescents consider 3/3 for diagnosis:

- A clinical diagnosis of oligomenorrhoea or amenorrhoea – menstrual cycles longer than 35 days or fewer than 10 periods a year.
- Clinical (hirsutism, acne, or androgen alopecia) or biochemical (raised free androgen index) evidence of hyperandrogenism.
- Polycystic ovaries on ultrasound examination.

Typical PCOS androgen profile

Plasma testosterone normal/high.
DHEAS normal.
SHBG low.
FSH low.
LH high.
LH:FSH >2 in 50%.
Prolactin slightly increased.

Hyperhidrosis

Important to differentiate between primary and secondary hyperhidrosis and investigate for causes of secondary hyperhidrosis as appropriate, including: infection, malignancy, carcinoid syndrome, hyperthyroidism, diabetes, medications, and pheochromocytoma. Treatment of primary hyperhidrosis depends on body site (see diagram below) and the availability of therapeutic options.

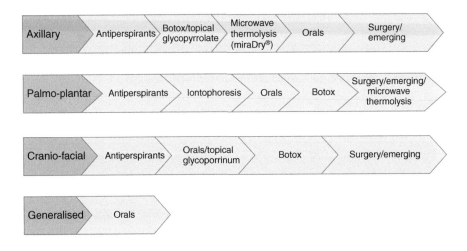

| Axillary | Antiperspirants | Botox/topical glycopyrrolate | Microwave thermolysis (miraDry®) | Orals | Surgery/emerging |

| Palmo-plantar | Antiperspirants | Iontophoresis | Orals | Botox | Surgery/emerging/microwave thermolysis |

| Cranio-facial | Antiperspirants | Orals/topical glycoporrinum | Botox | Surgery/emerging |

| Generalised | Orals |

Step 1

- **Aluminium chloride hexahydrate antiperspirant** [2]: various strengths (20% most frequently available). Should be applied to dry skin at night and washed off in morning. Irritation is common, and concurrent use of low-potency TCS is helpful.

Handbook of Skin Disease Management, First Edition. Zainab Jiyad and Carsten Flohr.
© 2023 John Wiley & Sons Ltd. Published 2023 by John Wiley & Sons Ltd.
Companion website: www.wiley.com/go/jiyad/handbookofskindiseasemanagement

Variable steps
as above

- **Botox** [4]: best for *axillary* hyperhidrosis. A RCT of 320 showed superiority over placebo, with 94% of treatment group responding at 4 weeks. Usually starch test performed first, 50–100 units onabotunlinumtoxinA injected into each axilla, typically 4–6 months apart. For palmoplantar, similar doses used into each palm/sole, but pain is a considerable limitation in this area.
- **Topical glycopyrrolate** [4]: 2 phase-3 RCTs of 344 and 353 participants showed superiority over placebo, for axillary hyperhidrosis. A non-randomised prospective study found 2% glycopyrrolate solution to be similarly efficacious to Botox injections. Not widely available.
- **Microwave thermolysis (miraDry®)** [4]: RCT of 120 participants with axillary hyperhidrosis using sham device, response rate of 89% in tx arm vs 54% in sham arm. Not widely available.
- **Iontophoresis** [4]: best for palmoplantar hyperhidrosis. RCT of 11 patients found a significant reduction in sweating, compared with placebo. Usually performed with tap water, some add a crushed anticholinergic tablet to treatment tray; in UK glycopyrronium bromide powder is available for this.
- **Orals** [4]: oxybutynin immediate-release 5mg 2–3 times/day or modified-release 5mg OD, increased by 5mg each week as necessary (max of 20mg); propantheline bromide less widely used – 15mg TDS, increase to max of 120mg/day; in USA oral glycopyrolate (1–2mg OD/BD) most widely used, not available in UK. In a SR, an average of 76.2% of patients improved with oral treatment. Dosages are limited by common unwanted side effects including dry mouth and urinary retention.

Surgery/
emerging

- **Surgery:** various techniques exist that include excision, curettage, liposuction for axillary hyperhidrosis. Sympathectomy is considered a last resort, and compensatory sweating can be an unwanted side effect.
- **Others:** ultrasound, fractional microneedle radiofrequency, laser treatment, subdermal laser procedures, PDT.

Ichthyosis

Categorised as syndromic vs non-syndromic ichthyoses (see below). Ichthyosis vulgaris and X-linked ichthyosis are the most common types and can be difficult to differentiate clinically.

Non-syndromic	**Onset in infancy or childhood:** ichthyosis vulgaris, X-linked ichthyosis.
	Autosomal recessive congenital ichthyoses (ARCIs): lamellar ichthyosis*, congenital ichthyosiform erythroderma*, harlequin ichthyosis, bathing suit ichthyosis, self-healing collodion baby*.
	Bullous ichthyoses.
Syndromic	Refsum, Netherton*, Sjogren-Larsson syndrome*, neutral lipid storage disease with ichthyosis*, trichothiodystrophy*.

* = causes of collodion baby (other causes: Gaucher, ectodermal dysplasias, Conradi-Hunermann-Happle syndrome).

X-linked and icthyosis vulgaris

- **Frequent emollients** [2].
- **Additional topical agents if needed** [2]: avoid in neonates and use with caution in small children: urea (various concentrations, use max 10%); lactic acid; salicylic acid (variable concentrations available, use higher strengths for stubborn areas); topical retinoids; propylene glycol.
- **Oral retinoids** [3]: rarely needed.

ARCIs

- **Neonatal intensive care** [4]: harlequin ichthyosis: intensive support addressing risks of poor feeding, dehydration, temperature imbalance, and skin infection. Neonatal collodion membrane: similar but less severe and may resolve within months.
- **Topicals, as above** [2]: bodysuit as used for eczema, worn under clothes, may be helpful.
- **Oral retinoids** [3]: harlequin ichthyosis – <u>acitretin, initially 0.5mg/kg/day, increasing to 1mg/kg/day if necessary.</u>
  <u>Not usually required for collodion baby, but may be indicated later.</u>
- **Vitamin D:** regular supplement required as ichthyosis predisposes to deficiency.
- **Biologics:** secukinumab appears promising in clinical trials.

Handbook of Skin Disease Management, First Edition. Zainab Jiyad and Carsten Flohr.
© 2023 John Wiley & Sons Ltd. Published 2023 by John Wiley & Sons Ltd.
Companion website: www.wiley.com/go/jiyad/handbookofskindiseasemanagement

General skin care

- **Bathing daily** recommended to loosen scales. Additives of sodium bicarbonate, antiseptics, bran, or rice starch can be helpful. Give patients clear instructions. Apply emollients straight after bathing.
- **Gentle rubbing** during bathing to help remove loose scale.
- **Scalp care:** Regular oily emollient such as coconut oil, keratolytic; fine-toothed comb to remove scales after washing.
- **Regular chiropody** for symptomatic palmoplantar keratoderma.
- **Check the ears** as clogging and hearing impairment can occur.
- **Ocular lubricants** and management of ectropion.

Infantile haemangioma (IH)

Management initially involves determining whether the IH is low risk or high risk (see below). However, each case needs to be individually assessed including discussion with parents, taking into account residua that may persist. Most proliferation occurs in first 6 months, and tx should ideally be initiated early to halt the proliferative process. Tx is not always necessary, and many just seek reassurance. *In general, treat uncomplicated IH with localised therapies. High-risk IHs are usually treated systemically.*

High risk:

- **Life-threatening:** 'beard area' IHs can be associated with airway haemangiomas. Sometimes, multiple IHs (5+) can be associated with liver haemangiomas, cardiac failure, and hypothyroidism.
- **Potential for functional impairment:** periorbital (visual impairment), lip/mouth (feeding impairment).
- **Potential for disfigurement:** face (any location but especially nose, lip, ear), breast in females, large/segmental IHs elsewhere.
- **Persistent ulceration:** areas prone to ulceration include perianal, gluteal, lips, columella, ear, intertriginous.
- **Syndromic:** PHACE = (P)osterior fossa and other structural brain malformations; large/segmental (H)aemangiomas of the face, neck, and/or scalp; anatomical anomalies of the cerebral or cervical (A)rteries; (C)ardiac anomalies/(C)oarctation of the aorta; and (E)ye abnormalities. LUMBAR = (L)ower body haemangioma; (U)rogenital abnormalities/(U)lceration; (M)yelopathy; (B)ony deformities; (A)no-rectal malformations/arterial anomalies; and (R)ectal anomalies.

Handbook of Skin Disease Management, First Edition. Zainab Jiyad and Carsten Flohr.
© 2023 John Wiley & Sons Ltd. Published 2023 by John Wiley & Sons Ltd.
Companion website: www.wiley.com/go/jiyad/handbookofskindiseasemanagement

Localised

- **Topical b-blockers** ①: use <u>timolol gel (ophthalmic) 0.5% BD</u> (particularly useful for superficial IH) until stable (6–12 months usually). Meta-analysis found pooled response rate of 83%. <u>Treatment of choice.</u> Can be trialled for telangiectatic residua too.
- **Potent/superpotent TCS** ③: OD. Use of these has been superseded by topical b-blockers, but they can be beneficial with ulcerated haemangiomas.
- **IL corticosteroids** ①: can be used for deep haemangiomas. In a retrospective review of 155 cases, 85% improved.

Systemic/ other

- **Oral propranolol** ①: network meta-analysis reported mean estimate of expected clearance of 95%. *Systemic of choice.* <u>See overleaf for dosing and initiation.</u>
- **Oral steroids** ①: superseded by oral propranolol but still used where propranolol is contraindicated/has failed. Mean expected clearance 43%. Sometimes used adjunctively with propranolol for tx-resistant cases. <u>2–3mg/kg.</u>
- **Rarely used:** vincristine, alpha-interferon, imiquimod, excision, embolisation, pulsed-dye laser.

Propanolol initiation: British Society for Paediatric Dermatology guidelines. Source: Adapted from Solman L, Glover M, Beattie PE, et al. Oral propranolol in the treatment of proliferating infantile haemangiomas: British Society for Paediatric Dermatology consensus guidelines. Br J Dermatol 2018;179(3):582–9.

Step 1

Check absolute contraindications:

1) Recent or ongoing hypoglycaemia.
2) Second-/third-degree heart block.
3) Hypersensitivity to propranolol.

If any of these are present – seek alternative tx.

Check relative contraindications:

1) Frequent wheezing.
2) Blood pressure not in normal age range.
3) Heart rate not in normal age range.

If any of these are present – treat in conjunction with paediatricians.

Step 2

Focused hx and examination:

1) Hx of loss of consciousness; maternal history of connective tissue disease; family hx of arrhythmia/sudden death.
2) Perform cardiovascular examination.
3) Check blood pressure and heart rate.
4) Check for segmental IH.

If any of above present, proceed as follows:

Obtain pre-treatment ECG IF:

- Heart rate below 5th percentile for age.
- Family hx of sudden death/arrythmia.
- Maternal history of connective tissue disease.

Obtain pre-treatment ECG and Echo IF:

- Bradycardia.
- Murmur identified.

IF cervicofacial segmental IH, perform following before initiating tx:

- ECG and Echo to be interpreted by cardiologist or paediatrician with cardiology interest.
- Brain MRI/MRA.

Step 3

Criteria for ambulatory propranolol:

1) Term birth and normal birthweight.
2) Older than 4 weeks.
3) No significant comorbidities.
4) Established feeds and appropriate weight gain.
5) Non-segmental IH.

If above met, initiate propranolol at dose of 1mg/kg daily in 3 divided doses. After at least 24 hrs, increase to 2mg/kg/day in 3 divided doses.

Review at 2–3 months:

1) Adjust the dose for weight (max 3mg/kg/day).
2) Stop tx if reduced oral intake or persistent wheezing.
3) Tx should extend beyond proliferative phase to avoid rebound growth.

Step 4

If criteria for ambulatory not met, admit to hospital to initiate propranolol.
See full guidelines for hospital monitoring requirements.

Keloid

It is important to establish the key issues and treatment goals of the patient at the outset: e.g. symptom relief, colour, scar size, functional issues. Realistic treatment expectations should be set.

Step 1

- **Potent/superpotent TCS** [2]: typically with occlusion (e.g steroid tape) is effective for thin/smaller lesions especially in children and the elderly.
- **Intralesional corticosteroids** [1]: used for thicker/larger lesions. Dose dependent on site and keloid size/firmness (2.5–40mg/mL), typically repeated every 4–6 weeks. Almost all patients have some response, but complete flattening only occurs in about 50% of those treated with steroids as monotherapy. Pre-treated with cryotherapy to soften the scar can help and work adjunctively to treat the keloid but risks hypopigmentation in dark skin.
- **Silicone sheets (e.g.Cica-care®)** [1]: a Cochrane review found a significant reduction in scar thickness. Most would use *as combination therapy*, rather than monotherapy.

Step 2

- **Intralesional 5-FU** [1]: a SR found 5-FU was effective in 45–96% of patients, based on 18 papers. The combination of intralesional steroids with 5-FU has been shown to perform better.
- **Laser** [3]: vascular lasers (PDL, Nd:YAG) are suitable for red, smaller lesions as mono- or combination therapy with intralesional treatment. Fractional CO_2 laser can be used for assisted drug delivery of steroids, and larger keloids can be shaved and cauterised with ablative CO_2 laser prior to adjuvant treatment.

Step 3

- **Excision with post-op therapies** [1]: excision technique and depth impact the high rate of recurrence, and surgery alone should be avoided. Commonly employed post-op therapies include radiotherapy (most effective especially for high recurrence risk sites and larger lesions), 1 or 2 adjuvant drugs (e.g. intralesional steroids, intralesional 5-FU), pressure, skin graft.

Handbook of Skin Disease Management, First Edition. Zainab Jiyad and Carsten Flohr.
© 2023 John Wiley & Sons Ltd. Published 2023 by John Wiley & Sons Ltd.
Companion website: www.wiley.com/go/jiyad/handbookofskindiseasemanagement

Refractory

- **Intralesional cryotherapy** [2]: can be effective at reducing keloid volume for primary keloids. Poor response for recurrent lesions and likely to cause hypopigmentation.
- **Intralesional bleomycin** [1]: recent meta-analysis found to be superior to IL steroids/5-FU. Electrochemotherapy increasingly used (general anaesthesia required).
- **Radiotherapy monotherapy** [3]: can be considered for keloids not responsive or too large for conventional therapy for symptom relief for up to 65% patients.

Combination treatments yield the best results, examples

Surgery + post-operative treatments; IL steroids + pressure therapy / silicone sheets; surgery + 5-FU; carbon dioxide laser + intralesional steroids; IL steroids + any treatment.

Keratosis pilaris (KP)

Frequently no treatment is necessary, but some may find benefit from treating inflammatory phases or where disease is more widespread. Counsel patients on realistic treatment outcomes and often limited improvement. KP differs from keratosis pilaris atrophicans, which encompasses a group of rare disorders that show atrophy and scarring in addition to keratotic papules – **see below for three variants of keratosis pilaris atrophicans.**

Ulerythema ophryogenes	Atrophoderma vermiculatum	Keratosis follicularis spinulosa decalvans
• Mainly affects eyebrows • Erythema and keratotic papules • Associated with a number of syndromes including Noonan and Rubinstein-Taybi syndrome	• Honeycomb depressions on the cheeks • Begins as erythema with keratotic papules • Associated with Rombo syndrome	• Scarring alopecia of scalp, eyebrows and eyelashes • Extensive KP changes across body

Step 1

- **Emollients and keratolytics** ③: emollients containing salicylic acid, urea, or lactic acid can reduce keratototic papules.
- **Topical retinoids** ②: a placebo-controlled RCT in 33 individuals found a significant improvement with topical tazoretene cream in pruritus, erythema, and roughness.
- **Topical steroids** ③: may be helpful in reducing erythema and symptoms. Use intermittently, bearing in mind the condition is life-long.

Step 2

- **Oral retinoids** ④: both isotretinoin and acitretin have been reported to be successful in case reports. Usually low-dose therapy is sufficient.

Refractory

- **Laser** ②: success with different laser therapies has been reported in a number of studies, including PDL, pulsed diode, IPL, Q-switched, and others.
- **Others:** tacrolimus, azelaic acid, calcipotriol, microdermabrasion.

Handbook of Skin Disease Management, First Edition. Zainab Jiyad and Carsten Flohr.
© 2023 John Wiley & Sons Ltd. Published 2023 by John Wiley & Sons Ltd.
Companion website: www.wiley.com/go/jiyad/handbookofskindiseasemanagement

Leg ulcers

The majority of leg ulcers are venous and managed in specialist clinics. Dedicated specialist nursing care is essential. Arterial ulcers should be referred to the vascular team, and diabetic (neuropathic) ulcers are managed in diabetic foot clinics. Less commonly, ulcers may be due to another underlying cause, which requires management of the underlying disease (see list on next page). Management of venous ulcers is outlined below. Lymphoedema is commonly present (see page 106).

Step 1

- **Wound care** [1]: *debride* necrotic tissue surgically or using autolytic dressings (e.g. alginates). Apply *dressings* that promote a moist environment (e.g. foams, hydrocolloids). *Minimise traumatic pressure.* Monitor for *infection* and treat when required.
- **Compression therapy** [1]: best evidence for multicomponent graduated bandaging. Obtaining ABPI and doppler waveforms can be considered before compression. Patients with ABPIs between 0.6 and 0.8 can have modified compression, but compression is contraindicated where ABPIs are <0.6. High-compression stockings are an alternative though there is less robust evidence.

Refractory

- **Consider biopsy:** to rule out malignancy or other causes.
- **Pentoxifylline** [1]: a meta-analysis of 11 trials found a significant effect when compared to placebo.
- **Dermal skin substitutes or cultured skin equivalents** [2].
- **Platelet-rich plasma** [1]: meta-analysis showed greater number of ulcers healed in tx group vs control group.
- **Hyperbaric oxygen** [1]: a Cochrane review and meta-analysis did not show any benefit at follow-up at 1 year.
- **Others:** flavonoids, aspirin, mesoglycan, sulodexide, prostaglandins, honey, surgery for incompetent veins, growth factors.

Handbook of Skin Disease Management, First Edition. Zainab Jiyad and Carsten Flohr.
© 2023 John Wiley & Sons Ltd. Published 2023 by John Wiley & Sons Ltd.
Companion website: www.wiley.com/go/jiyad/handbookofskindiseasemanagement

Causes

- Venous
- Arterial/arterio-venous
- Neuropathic (including diabetic)
- Pressure
- Pyoderma gangrenosum
- Malignancy
- Infections (e.g. buruli ulcer)
- Marjolin's ulcer
- Connective-tissue diseases
- Vasculitis
- Vasculopathy (micro-occlusive)
- Martorell's ulcer (hypertensive ulcer)
- Sickle-cell disease
- Calciphylaxis
- Necrobiosis lipoidica
- Necrotising fasciitis
- Hydroxyurea ulcers
- Panniculitides

Lentigo maligna (LM)

The challenges of LM lie in its propensity to extend beyond clinically obvious margins, its potentially indolent nature, its occurrence in older persons with multiple comorbidities, and its development on a cosmetically sensitive site. Confocal microscopy can be useful in delineating margins. Treatment options are presented here in order of what is most commonly used.

> **Active surveillance** of lentigo maligna is a valid treatment option. The decision on which treatment pathway to take requires a clear discussion with the patient, detailing risks and benefits.

Option 1

- **Surgical excision - WLE** [3]: most commonly used. Most guidelines recommend 5–10mm margins of excision.
- **Mohs micrographic surgery (MMS)** [3]: 'slow Mohs' using fixed formalin sections is often preferred because frozen sections can be difficult to interpret. In a retrospective study of 423 LM lesions, recurrence rates were higher in wide excision group (5.9%) vs MMS group (1.9%).

Option 2

- **Imiquimod 5%** [4]: SR of 471 patients reported clearance rate of 78.3%. Wide variety of tx schedules used but SR concluded that 6–7 applications of imiquimod per week, with at least 60 applications, showed the greatest odds of complete clinical and histological clearance.

Option 3

- **Radiotherapy** [3]: where surgery is not feasible (cosmetic outcome, comorbidities). SR reported mean recurrence rate of 11.5% based on crude analysis of 454 patients.

Other options

- **Active surveillance, as above:** the risk of transformation into melanoma <5%.
- **Not currently recommended:** cryotherapy /curettage and cautery. Laser ablation – in a retrospective study, 1 of 15 patients (6.7%) suffered recurrence following CO_2 laser ablation, very limited evidence at this stage.

Handbook of Skin Disease Management, First Edition. Zainab Jiyad and Carsten Flohr.
© 2023 John Wiley & Sons Ltd. Published 2023 by John Wiley & Sons Ltd.
Companion website: www.wiley.com/go/jiyad/handbookofskindiseasemanagement

Lichen planopilaris (LPP)

Explain that the **aim** is to treat active disease to prevent further hair loss and that scarred, 'burnt out' areas, will usually not be reversible.

Active disease is suggested by:

- Symptoms (itching, pain, burning).
- Perifollicular hyperkeratosis and perifollicular erythema.
- Ongoing hair loss.
- Active disease on biopsy.

All Patients

1) **Biopsy:** scarring alopecia biopsy protocol (page 217).
2) Take **baseline photographs.**
3) Recommend **hair camouflage** (see Appendix D)/wigs.

At any stage consider tapering course of **oral steroids** (0.5–1mg/kg) to stabilise active disease.

Step 1

- **Potent/superpotent TCS** ③: use OD/BD to active areas and taper as improves.
- **AND/OR IL corticosteroid** ③: injections (10mg/mL, consider reducing to 5mg/mL for frontal scalp) to active edge, every 4–6 weeks.
- Treat any concurrent **androgenetic alopecia** (see pages 57 and 109).

Step 2

- **Hydroxychloroquine** ②: all but mild cases should be initiated on 5mg/kg, if tolerated (for 300mg, do 200/400mg alternating dose daily). A 2018 SR found a global response rate of 51% of 127 included patients.

Handbook of Skin Disease Management, First Edition. Zainab Jiyad and Carsten Flohr.
© 2023 John Wiley & Sons Ltd. Published 2023 by John Wiley & Sons Ltd.
Companion website: www.wiley.com/go/jiyad/handbookofskindiseasemanagement

Lichen planopilaris (LPP)

Step 3

- **Methotrexate** ②: RCT of MTX <u>15mg/weekly</u> vs hydroxychloroquine of 29 patients for 6 months found MTX was more effective in decreasing Lichen Planopilaris Activity Index (LPPAI).

Refractory

- **Limited evidence:** Ciclosporin ④ (<u>3–5mg/kg;</u> evidence from case series reports: 10 out of 13 patients in 1 series improved), MMF ③ (<u>0.5–1g BD</u>; meta-analysis found pooled complete/partial response of 70%), pioglitazone ④ (<u>15mg/day</u>), azathioprine, JAK inhibitors.
- **Very limited evidence:** griseofulvin, oral retinoids, thalidomide, naltrexone, excimer laser, tetracyclines, antihistamines.

A biopsy is often undertaken to confirm the diagnosis. An association with hepatitis C has been shown in some but not all populations. Some recommend testing for hep C as routine, but most would err on screening for risk factors first. Prognostically, most cases of cutaneous LP will resolve within 1–2 years. Mucosal involvement tends to be chronic. Particular subtypes of LP will respond to other therapies, e.g. TCS with occlusions/IL steroids in hypertrophic LP. The treatment of nail disease can be particularly challenging – *see overleaf.*

Step 1

- **Potent/superpotent topical corticosteroids** [2]: often this is all that is required for localised disease. Used adjunctively in widespread disease. Evidence from RCTs for oral LP. Tacrolimus is recommended alternative in cases of oral LP, but limited efficacy for cutaneous disease. IL steroids for resistant disease/areas.
- **Oral corticosteroids** [2]: generally 30–40mg used as starting dose with gradual wean over several weeks. In some patients, this will ensure resolution. However, others will relapse and require one of the treatments below. In a comparative study of oral steroids vs topical for oral LP, similar clinical responses were noted in both groups.

Step 2

- **Phototherapy** [3]: usually NBUVB is used, but PUVA is alternative. A retrospective review of 50 patients found that a complete response was achieved in 70% of patients treated with UVB. Further comparative study of PUVA vs NBUVB for LP found no difference in response.
- **Acitretin** [4]: multicenter RCT of 65 patients found 64% of those treated with acitretin 30mg/day for 8 weeks improved, which was significant compared with placebo. Start at 25mg OD and titrate as needed, see page 191.
- **Methotrexate** [4]: a comparative study of MTX vs oral steroid found no significant difference between the 2 groups and that 63 of 79 patients treated with MTX improved.

Refractory

- **Case reports/most used:** ciclosporin [3], dapsone [2], hydroxychloroquine [2], MMF [4].
- **Others:** thalidomide, apremilast, azathioprine, biologics.

Handbook of Skin Disease Management, First Edition. Zainab Jiyad and Carsten Flohr.
© 2023 John Wiley & Sons Ltd. Published 2023 by John Wiley & Sons Ltd.
Companion website: www.wiley.com/go/jiyad/handbookofskindiseasemanagement

Nail LP

1) **Topicals**
   TCS as ointment/cream.
2) **Steroid (triamcinolone) injections**
   Usually <u>2.5–10mg/mL</u>. **Pain** is a limiting factor, and whilst nerve blocks can be used, rapid treatment is reported with concurrent coolant analgesia, vibrating devices, or ethyl chloride spray, even in adolescents. This diagram illustrates a widely used technique with injections into four periungual sites, to ensure symmetrical delivery to the nail matrix and bed.

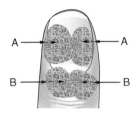

3) **Oral retinoids**
   Retinoids are considered second-line for nail disease, with **acitretin** being most commonly used. Case reports support **alitretinoin** as alternative.
4) **Others**
   Ciclosporin, azathioprine, and MMF may produce some benefit in refractory cases. 6-month courses minimise side effects, as nail disease tends to be slow to relapse. **Methotrexate** has conflicting reports. **Oral CS** sometimes used where multiple nails affected. Rare reports of **biologics (etanercept).**

LP, psoriasis, or 20-nail dystrophy?

Differentiating LP of the nails from psoriasis of the nails can be difficult. Trachyonychia, which describes rough longitudinal ridging with thickening of the nails and distal brittleness, is common in both conditions. When all 20 digits are affected by trachyonychia, the term '20-nail dystrophy' has previously been used. Although there may be no underlying cause for trachyonychia, psoriasis and LP are common culprits, and skin examination and hx should screen for these conditions in particular.

Favours LP	Common to both LP or psoriasis	Favours psoriasis
Longitudinal splits in nail		
Pterygium		Oily spots
	Onycholysis	Scaling of nail fold
	Discolouration	Pustules
	Subungual hyperkeratosis	
	Nail loss	
	Nail plate thickening	
	Pitting	
	Altered nail shape or curvature	

Lichen sclerosus (LS) – genital

Often, but not always, a *biopsy* is undertaken to confirm the diagnosis. Enquire about **i)** primary symptoms (e.g. itch), **ii)** sexual dysfunction, **iii)** urinary dysfunction (more common in men, rare in women). Some may require referral to urology/urogynaecology/psychosexual clinic. Explain that this is a chronic disease and treatment is titrated to maintain control of symptoms and may be required long term. The risk of SCC is very low in well-managed disease. Once disease is stable, patients can be discharged with a management plan and advised on when to seek help if symptoms are not responding to usual treatment.

Step 1

Initiate following and review at 3 months (to assess response to treatment) if confident and experienced in the management of LS. All children should be referred to a specialist to start treatment:

- **Superpotent TCS** [1]: OD for 1 month, then alternate days for 1 month, then twice weekly for 1 month. Advise patients to use approximately half a fingertip unit. The aim is to induce remission before moving into maintenance phase. Potent TCS commonly used in children.
- **Moisturiser + soap substitute** [4]: essential adjunctive treatments. Ointments are preferred; however, key is to find one that suits the patient to ensure regular use.

Step 2

- **Check compliance, consider malignancy, re-evaluate diagnosis, and refer to specialist – for males, if there is no response after 1–3 months, refer to urologists for circumcision.**

The following only applies to female patients as males are referred for circumcision:

- **Superpotent TCS maintenance regimen** [1]: once or twice weekly, as above.
- **Topical calcineurin inhibitors** [4]: found to be inferior to TCS in RCTs. Not recommended in most guidelines, but may have a role in treating children with LS or for maintenance. Risk of potentiating malignancy.

Refractory

Refractory cases should be referred to a specialist, particularly to re-evaluate the diagnosis, as LS is usually responsive to treatment if managed as above.

- **Not recommended:** topical hormonal treatments, laser treatment.

Handbook of Skin Disease Management, First Edition. Zainab Jiyad and Carsten Flohr.
© 2023 John Wiley & Sons Ltd. Published 2023 by John Wiley & Sons Ltd.
Companion website: www.wiley.com/go/jiyad/handbookofskindiseasemanagement

Linear IgA disease

Occurs in both adults and children, where it has previously been termed chronic bullous disease of childhood.

All Patients

1) **Skin biopsy for histology (lesional skin) and direct IMF (perilesional):** see page 218.
2) **Check drug history:** vancomycin is particularly implicated. Other causes include NSAIDs, captopril, phenytoin, lithium.

Course of oral steroids can be used for severe flares, e.g. 20–40mg as reducing regimen over a few weeks.

Step 1

- **Dapsone** ③: *see page 186 for initiation.*
- **Topical steroids** ④: use as adjunctive therapy, except where there is minimal disease.

Step 2

- **Sulfonamides** ④: sulfapyridine, not easily available. *Use 500mg TDS, maximum of 6g. Or sulfasalazine 500mg BD-QDS.* Higher doses 1g QDS can be used, as per inflammatory bowel diseases doses. Sulfamethoxypyridine is not easily available but can be *used in doses of 0.25–1.5g/day.*
- **Colchicine** ④: *500 micrograms start at OD and increase to BD after 1 week, as tolerated, to maximum of 2mg.*

Refractory

- **MMF** ④: *see page 188 for initiation and dosing.*
- **Ciclosporin** ④: *see page 183 for initiation and dosing.*
- **Azathioprine** ④: *see page 185 for initiation and dosing.*
- **Others:** rituximab, IVIG, tetracycline +/− nicotinamide, anti-TNF, erythromycin, thalidomide.

Handbook of Skin Disease Management, First Edition. Zainab Jiyad and Carsten Flohr.
© 2023 John Wiley & Sons Ltd. Published 2023 by John Wiley & Sons Ltd.
Companion website: www.wiley.com/go/jiyad/handbookofskindiseasemanagement

Lipodermatosclerosis (LDS)

Treatment of venous disease, which is the underlying cause in the majority of cases, is key.

All Patients

1) **Focused history** screening for underlying cause and exacerbating factors.
2) **Consider doppler studies/ABPIs** if compression planned.
3) Treat venous disease and lymphoedema: **elevation, exercise, weight management, and skin care.**

Step 1

- **Compression** [4]: usually treatment begins with compression bandaging before maintenance with compression garments (see page 107).
- **TCS** [4]: moderate potency–potent TCS can sometimes alleviate the pain associated with acute LDS

Step 2

- **Anabolic steroids** [2]: a crossover study of 23 patients that compared compression with placebo vs compression with stanozolol found that the rate of healing when patients took stanozolol was double that of placebo, and this was assumed to be biologically important. Stanozolol availability is limited, consider danazol at a dose of 100–200mg BD as alternative. May be particularly useful for treating acute exacerbations to enable resumption of compression. Oxandrolone is alternative.
- **Pentoxifylline** [4]: doses of 400mg BD-TDS.
- **Topical capsaicin** [4]: trial daily for 3–4 weeks, as tolerated.

Refractory

- **Intralesional steroids** [3]: in a review of 26 patients who had IL steroids with compression alleviated pain in all but one.
- **Surgery** [4]: very rarely employed and unlikely to be successful.

Often, acute exacerbations of LDS are mistaken for **cellulitis**. Although similar features are shared (a red, painful leg), the key differentiating feature is the absence of systemic symptoms (e.g. fever, lethargy, malaise) in LDS.

Handbook of Skin Disease Management, First Edition. Zainab Jiyad and Carsten Flohr.
© 2023 John Wiley & Sons Ltd. Published 2023 by John Wiley & Sons Ltd.
Companion website: www.wiley.com/go/jiyad/handbookofskindiseasemanagement

Lupus erythematosus (LE)

Treatment varies depending on the subtype and systemic involvement. Discoid lupus is a scarring disease, and treatment should be aggressive to prevent disfigurement. **Use weaning systemic steroids 0.5–1mg/kg if widespread/severe/ rapidly progressive.**

All Patients

1) **Check drug history:** see next page for causes of drug-induced SCLE.
2) **Screen for symptoms of systemic disease (SLE):** see next page for classification criteria.
3) **Recommend sun protection and advise smoking cessation.**
4) **Investigations:** FBC, U/E, LFTs, CRP/ESR, ANA, ENAs, immunoglobulins, complement, urine dip +/- PCR, skin biopsy+IMF.

Step 1

- **Potent/superpotent TCS** [4]: use OD/BD. Use for active disease only – e.g. erythema, scale, itch, etc. IL steroids can be used for areas resistant to TCS. Typically 2.5–5mg/ mL and 0.1ml per 1 cm².
- **Topical tacrolimus 0.1% ointment** [4]: use OD/BD. Pimecrolimus has also been used in studies

Step 2

- **Hydroxychloroquine** [4]: 200mg OD or BD (max 5mg/kg), change brands if intolerant. In a review of 1002 patients, 81.5% of those treated with hydroxychloroquine improved.

Step 3

- **Add quinacrine** [3]: 100mg OD. In a retrospective review of 34 patients who did not respond to hydroxychloroquine monotherapy, adding quinacrine resulted in 84% response rate. Use as monotherapy in those with concerns re: ocular toxicity.

Handbook of Skin Disease Management, First Edition. Zainab Jiyad and Carsten Flohr.
© 2023 John Wiley & Sons Ltd. Published 2023 by John Wiley & Sons Ltd.
Companion website: www.wiley.com/go/jiyad/handbookofskindiseasemanagement

> **Step 4**

- **Methotrexate** [4]: placebo-controlled RCTs show efficacy. A retrospective review of 43 patients treated with MTX found improvement in all but one. See page 181 for dosage and initiation.

> **Refractory**

First-line for refractory disease:
- **Retinoids** [4]: in RCT comparing hydroxychloroquine, 46% of 28 treated with 50mg/day acitretin responded. Some evidence for isotretinoin and alitretinoin too. Dosing: see appendix A.
- **Dapsone** [3]: in a retrospective review of 33, 16 showed partial–excellent improvement. Standard dose: see page 186.
- **MMF** [3]: in a prospective study of 10, a significant reduction in CLASI was seen. Standard dose: see page 188.

Second-line: thalidomide [1] (50–200mg/day).

Third-line: azathioprine [3], CsA [4], belimumab [4], IVIG [3], rituximab [3], cyclophosphamide [3], UVA-1 [4].

Drug causes SCLE – descending order of reported frequency:

Antihypertensives (calcium channel blockers, ACE inhibitors, diuretics, b-blockers)
Proton pump inhibitors
Antifungals (terbinafine and griseofulvin)
Chemotherapeutics
Immunomodulators (leflunomide, interferon, hydroxychloroquine)
Biologics
Antihistamines
Antibiotics (minocycline, doxycycline)
Antiepileptics
NSAIDs
Other

Association with SLE:

Acute CLE >90%
SCLE 50%
Generalised DLE 15–28%
Chilblain lupus 20–25%
Localised DLE 5–10%
Lupus panniculitis 5–10%
Lupus tumidus – rare

ANA positivity (1:80 titre):

Acute CLE 97%
SCLE 71%
DLE 20–48%
Lupus panniculitis 44%
Lupus tumidus 25%

Lupus antibodies

dsDNA – nephritis	**Ro** – SCLE (75–90%)	**ssDNA** – risk of SLE in DLE
Sm – lupus specific	**La** – SCLE (30–40%)	**rRNP** – neuropsychiatric
U1RNP – mixed CTD	**Histone** – drug-induced LE	**C1q** – severe SLE + lupus nephritis

2019 EULAR/ACR Lupus Erythematosus Classification Criteria: ANA ≥ 1:80 is essential

Constitutional
- fever (2 points)

Haematological
- leukopenia (3 points)
- thrombocytopenia (4 points)
- autoimmune haemolysis (4 points)

Neuropsychiatric
- delirium (2 points)
- psychosis (3 points)
- seizure (5 points)

Musculoskeletal
- joint involvement (6 points)

Mucocutaneous
- non-scarring alopecia (2 points)
- oral ulcers (2 points)

- SCLE/DLE (4 points)
- ACLE (6 points)

Serosal
- pleural/pericardial effusion (5 points)
- acute pericarditis (6 points)

Renal
- proteinuria (>0.5g/24h) (4 points)
- renal bx class II/V lupus nephritis (8 points)
- renal bx class III/IV lupus nephritis (10 points)

Antiphospholipid antibodies
- anti-cardiolipin/B2GP1/ lupus anticoagulant (2 points)

Complement proteins
- low C3 OR low C4 (3 points)
- low C3 AND low C4 (4 points)

SLE-specific antibodies
- anti-dsDNA or anti-Smith (6 points)

A score of 10+ (with at least 1 clinical criteria) is required (only the highest-weighted criteria within each domain is counted).

Lymphoedema

Broadly, lymphoedema is classified as either primary or secondary. Patients with primary lymphoedema are born with a genetically determined lymphatic anomaly, whilst secondary lymphoedema occurs as a result of extrinsic damage. Rarely is a reversible cause identified (see page 212 for causes), and generally the aim of treatment is to reduce swelling and prevent progression and complications.

All Patients

1) **Focused history screening** for underlying cause and exacerbating factors.
2) **Encourage mobilisation/gradual exercise.**
3) Manage **obesity.**
4) Mobilisation preferred state, but encourage **elevation** when lying/sitting in armchair.
5) Meticulous **skin hygiene** and treat any fungal disease.
6) Consider **ABPIs/Dopplers,** prior to compression.

With moderate–severe disease, combined decongestive therapy is employed: this is a combination treatment of compression, manual lymphatic drainage (only in select cases, evidence for this limited), exercise, and skin care.

Step 1

- **Compression** ③: usually treatment begins with compression bandaging before maintenance with compression garments (see overleaf).

Step 2

- **Manual lymphatic drainage (MLD)** ③: performed by experienced therapists. A Cochrane review concluded there was evidence to suggest that MLD may offer additional benefit to compression bandaging, following breast cancer tx. However, *evidence for MLD is limited overall.* Visit www.mlduk.org.uk for a list of accredited therapists worldwide.

Handbook of Skin Disease Management, First Edition. Zainab Jiyad and Carsten Flohr.
© 2023 John Wiley & Sons Ltd. Published 2023 by John Wiley & Sons Ltd.
Companion website: www.wiley.com/go/jiyad/handbookofskindiseasemanagement

> Refractory

- **Intermittent pneumatic compression** ②: limited evidence, experience shows many derive no benefit.
- **Debulking surgery:** rarely used as poor results, but can be used for genital lymphoedema. **Liposuction** can be helpful for select cases of treatment-resistant limb lymphoedema.

Patients with lymphoedema are at risk of **cellulitis**. If they experience two or more episodes of cellulitis per year, consider long-term prophylactic phenoxy-methylpenicillin (Pen V) at dose of 250mg twice daily (or 500mg twice daily if BMI > 33).

Compression wraps (velcro wraps)

- **Best for:** bulky heavy legs, shape distortion, dependency, limited mobility, compromised skin integrity, unable to don traditional hosiery, easier for carers to apply, lipodermatosclerosis, elderly patients.
- **Options:** wraps come in sections – separate foot, calf, knee, thigh sections.
- **How and what to prescribe:** various manufacturers, use www.hadhealth.com to guide selection – select 'products' and choose 'EasyWraps®' and follow guidance for upper/lower limb and measuring tips.
- **Limitations/contraindications:** severe limb shape distortion, severely compromised skin integrity, DVT.

Compression bandaging

- **Best for:** wet legs (active lymphorrhea), wounds, severe shape distortion, pain, frail patients, lipodermatosclerosis, heavily excess volumes.
- **Options:** Tubifast® liners, under-cast padding (Soffban®), short stretch cohesive bandages (Actico®)
- **How:** needs to be performed by nurse qualified in performing compression bandaging.
- **Limitations/contraindications:** lack of follow-up availability with nurse to change bandages, DVT.

Compression stockings

- **Best for:** normal leg shape, skin intact, patient able to bend to apply, best if ambulatory.
- **Options:** below knee/above knee, 4 choices of compression class (see table below), open or closed toe, grip top if not allergic to silicon (to hold stocking).
- **How and what to prescribe:** various manufacturers. Can download 'Juzo Care App' on smartphone, choose 'health professional', select 'choose a lower leg garment for my patient' and follow the guidance to the right product, which you can prescribe.
- **Limitations/contraindications:** mild/moderate limb shape distortion, wet/leaking legs, wounds, gross swelling, patient cannot bend to don/doff, arterial disease, avoid if using greasy emollients, DVT.

Compression stocking classifications in mmHg

Standard	Class 1	Class 2	Class 3	Class 4
British	14–17	18–24	25–35	N/A
European	15–21	23–32	34–46	>49
USA	15–20	20–30	30–40	N/A

Male pattern hair loss

All Patients

1) **Bloods:** evidence limited but usually recommended that ferritin levels are >70. Some dermatologists recommend checking and correcting B12, folate + TFTs as well.
2) Take **baseline photographs.**
3) Recommend **hair camouflage** (see Appendix D)/wigs.

Step 1

- **Topical minoxidil** [1]: evidence suggests that 5% BD is more effective. Foam preparation has no propylene glycol, which can cause irritation. Treat for at least 4 months before assessing efficacy; hair shedding in first 6 weeks of use can occur. Hair loss resumes on discontinuation, so treatment should continue indefinitely.

Step 2

- **Finasteride** [1]: meta-analysis showed at up to 12 months of treatment, the mean percentage change in hair count was 9% higher in those treated with finasteride compared with placebo. Prescribe 1mg/day. Continue for at least 12 months.

Step 3

- **Low-level laser light therapy (LLLT)** [2]: RCT of 128 males LLLT vs sham device found mean terminal hair count increase of 18–26 per cm^2 in active treatment. Generally used as *adjunctive* treatment. Patient purchases product for home use and follows instructions of device.
- **Hair transplantation:** mainstay of surgical treatment in patients with good donor hair. Continuing finasteride following transplantation achieves better long-term results.
- **Emerging treatments:** microneedling, mesotherapy, platelet-rich plasma, oral minoxidil, intralesional dutasteride, topical 5α reductase inhibitors.

Handbook of Skin Disease Management, First Edition. Zainab Jiyad and Carsten Flohr.
© 2023 John Wiley & Sons Ltd. Published 2023 by John Wiley & Sons Ltd.
Companion website: www.wiley.com/go/jiyad/handbookofskindiseasemanagement

Mastocytosis of the skin

Mastocytosis with skin lesions may be limited to the skin (cutaneous mastocytosis) or systemic.

All Patients

1) **Take history screening for systemic mast cell mediator release:** flushing, wheezing, diarrhoea, abdominal pain, fatigue.
2) **Advise avoidance of triggers, including:** extremes of weather, alcohol, exercise, stress, opioids, aspirin, NSAIDs.
3) **Patients with suspected systemic disease should be referred to a specialist centre (dermatology/haematology).**
4) **With the exception of solitary mastocytoma, perform blood tests to screen for systemic involvement:** FBC, tryptase level (>20 ng/mL abnormal), LFTs, vitamin D, IgE with ImmunoCAP for bee and wasp venom sensitisation. Peripheral blood KIT mutation sequencing for D816V is becoming standard practice for adults with skin lesions.
5) **Do a baseline DEXA for all adults with repeat examination every 3–5 years for those with systemic disease.**
6) **Consider EpiPen for children with extensive skin involvement and all adults.**

Solitary mastocytoma

<u>Usually no treatment is required, other than avoidance of mast cell degranulation triggers.</u>
- **Regular H1 antihistamines** [4]: may be valuable for children with associated flushing or blistering.
- **Potent TCS** [3]: in a study of 130 patients, resolution was faster in those treated with TCS (16.4 months) vs those untreated (37.5 months), although no difference in number of resolved lesions. <u>OD/BD 6 weeks.</u>
- **Surgical excision** [4]: case reports of this being performed, in exceptional cases.

Handbook of Skin Disease Management, First Edition. Zainab Jiyad and Carsten Flohr.
© 2023 John Wiley & Sons Ltd. Published 2023 by John Wiley & Sons Ltd.
Companion website: www.wiley.com/go/jiyad/handbookofskindiseasemanagement

MPCM (UP)/
diffuse cutaneous
mastocytosis/
TMEP

- **Antihistamines** [4]: non-sedating H1 antihistamines are used first-line for those with symptoms of flushing, burning, and itch, *titrated as necessary to max QDS*. H2 antihistamines can be added and are suggested to be more beneficial for abdominal pain, hyperacidity, and diarrhoea.
- **Moderate–ultrapotent TCS** [3]: short-term use in limited areas in adults can improve the appearance of UP. Skin lesions improved with TCS and occlusion in one study. OD/BD 6 weeks.
- **Sodium cromoglycate** [4]: branded topical preparations are not available but extemporaneous mixtures can be produced between 1 and 4%, usually applied BD. Oral cromoglycate has been shown to improve pruritus and whealing as well as gastrointestinal symptoms – 200mg QDS in over 14 years old; 100mg QDS for children aged 2–13 years.
- **Phototherapy** [3]: both PUVA and NBUVB have shown short-term benefit on pruritus and appearance. In a retrospective review, improvement was seen in 14 of 20 UP patients treated with PUVA.
- **Other** [4]: ketotifen (esp. if GI symptoms), oral steroids (for severe flares), montelukast, alpha interferon. Adrenaline for all adults and children with extensive skin lesions

Melanoma

Management rests on determining the stage of melanoma, *see below*. Advanced disease is not discussed here as this should be undertaken in conjunction with oncologists with experience of managing advanced melanoma. Lentigo maligna is a challenging entity, and treatment of this is discussed separately (*see page 94*).

Melanoma management overview

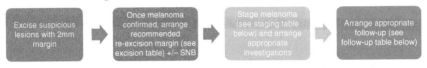

Step 1 – MDT discussion and clinical staging (AJCC) usually undertaken at this point. Re-excise with recommended margins +/– sentinel node biopsy

Melanoma excision margin recommendations – British, American, and European

Breslow thickness	Excision margins UK (BAD)	Excision margins USA (AAD)	Excision margins European (EORTC)
In-situ	0.5cm	0.5–1cm	0.5cm
<1mm	1cm	1cm	1cm
1.01–2mm	1–2cm	1–2cm	1cm
2.1–4mm	2–3cm	2cm	2cm
>4mm	3cm	2cm	2cm

Sentinel node biopsy? UK (NICE) guidelines do not recommend SNB in stage IA, and for Breslow 0.8–1mm, it can be considered if there is ulceration, lymphovascular invasion, or mitotic index 2 or more. Updated AJCC guidelines recommend SNB in T1b or higher (which includes BT <1mm), as do European clinical practice guidelines (ESMO, EORTC, EDF).

Handbook of Skin Disease Management, First Edition. Zainab Jiyad and Carsten Flohr.
© 2023 John Wiley & Sons Ltd. Published 2023 by John Wiley & Sons Ltd.
Companion website: www.wiley.com/go/jiyad/handbookofskindiseasemanagement

AJCC TNM eighth edition staging system of melanoma

Primary tumour (T)	Lymph nodes (N)	Metastases (M)
TX primary tumour thickness cannot be assessed **T0** no evidence of primary tumour **Tis** melanoma in-situ	**NX** regional nodes not assessed **N0** no regional metastases	**M0** no evidence of distant metastases

T1 ≤1.0mm unknown/ unspecified ulceration
  T1a <0.8mm without ulceration
  T1b <0.8mm with ulceration OR 0.8–1mm with or without ulceration
	N1 1 tumour-involved node or in-transit, satellite, and/or microsatellite metastases with no tumour-involved nodes
	  N1a 1 clinically occult (i.e. detected by SLN biopsy)
	  N1b 1 clinically detected
	  N1c no regional lymph node disease but in-transit/satellite/ microsatellite metastases
		M1 evidence of distant metastasis
		  M1a(0) distant metastasis to skin, soft tissue including muscle, and/or non-regional lymph node, <u>normal LDH</u>
		  M1a(1) distant metastasis to skin, soft tissue including muscle, and/or non-regional lymph node, <u>elevated LDH</u>

T2 >1–2mm unknown/ unspecified ulceration
  T2a >1–2mm without ulceration
  T2b >1–2mm with ulceration
	N2 2 or 3 tumour-involved nodes or in-transit, satellite, and/or microsatellite metastases with 1 tumour-involved node
	  N2a 2 or 3 clinically occult (i.e. detected by SLN biopsy)
	  N1b 2 or 3, at least 1 of which was clinically detected
	  N2c 1 clinically occult or clinically detected and in-transit/ satellite/ microsatellite metastases
		M1b distant metastasis to lung with or without M1a sites of disease
		  M1b(0) as above, normal LDH
		  M1b(1) as above, elevated LDH

T3 >2–4mm unknown/unspecified ulceration
  T3a >2–4mm without ulceration
  T3b >2–4mm with ulceration
	N3 4 or more tumour-involved nodes or in-transit, satellite, and/or microsatellite metastases with 2 or more tumour-involved nodes, or any number of matted nodes without or with in-transit, satellite, and/or microsatellite metastases
	  N3a 4 or more clinically occult (i.e. detected by SLN biopsy)
	  N3b 4 or more, at least 1 of which was clinically detected, or presence of any number of matted nodes
	  N3c 2 or more clinically occult or clinically detected and/or presence of any number of matted nodes
		M1c distant metastasis to non-CNS visceral sites with or without M1a or M1b sites of disease
		  M1c(0) as above, normal LDH
		  M1c(1) as above, elevated LDH

Primary tumour (T)	Lymph nodes (N)	Metastases (M)
T4 >4mm unknown/ unspecified ulceration **T4a** >4mm without ulceration **T4b** >4mm with ulceration		**M1d** distant metastasis to CNS with or without M1a, M1b, or M1c sites of disease **M1d(0)** as above, normal LDH **M1d(1)** as above, elevated LDH

Source: Amin MB, Edge SB, Greene FL, et al, eds. AJCC Cancer Staging Manual. 8th ed. New York: Springer; 2017.

Pathological staging of melanoma, AJCC

Where T is...	Where N is...	Where M is...	Then pathological stage is:
Tis	N0	M0	**0**
T1a	N0	M0	**IA**
T1b	N0	M0	**IA**
T2a	N0	M0	**IB**
T2b	N0	M0	**IIA**
T3a	N0	M0	**IIA**
T3b	N0	M0	**IIB**
T4a	N0	M0	**IIB**
T4b	N0	M0	**IIC**
T0	N1b, N1c	M0	**IIIB**
T0	N2b, N2c, N3b, or N3c	M0	**IIIC**
T1a/b-T2a	N1a or N2a	M0	**IIIA**
T1a/b-T2a	N1b/c or N2b	M0	**IIIB**
T2b/T3a	N1a-N2b	M0	**IIIB**
T1a-T3a	N2c or N3a/b/c	M0	**IIIC**
T3b/T4a	Any N ≥N1	M0	**IIIC**
T4b	N1a-N2c	M0	**IIIC**
T4b	N3a/b/c	M0	**IIID**
Any T, Tis	Any N	M1	**IV**

Source: Amin MB, Edge SB, Greene FL, et al, eds. AJCC Cancer Staging Manual. 8th ed. New York: Springer; 2017.

Which investigations?

- **Gene expression profiling and proteomics:** NICE recommends consideration of BRAF analysis in stages IIA and higher. Specifically, they recommend immunohistochemistry as the first test for BRAF V600E, if available.
- **Check vitamin D levels (NICE) in all patients.**
- **Check LDH and baseline bloods:** usually performed in stage III and above.
- **Staging imaging:** NICE recommendations are to consider staging with whole-body and brain contrast-enhanced (CE)-CT for people with stage IIB melanoma; for IIC-IV offer staging with whole-body and brain CE-CT. NICE do specify MRI brain is preferable if available.
- **Whole-body MRI:** offered to children/young persons (0-24 years) and pregnant women with stage IIB-IV disease (NICE).

Melanoma: assessment and management. NICE guideline [Internet]. 2022 [cited 2022 Sep 13]. Available from: www.nice.org.uk/guidance/ng14.

Melasma

Medical photography is crucial to monitor and track changes as they are often gradual and subtle, which may lead to a treatment being incorrectly labelled as ineffective. Camouflage services should be offered.

> Photoprotection to UV and visible light for patients with skin of colour is essential. The evidence suggests that melasma can be both prevented and improved with regular application.

Step 1

- **Triple combination cream** [4]: tx of choice. These combine a hydroquinone, a steroid, and a topical retinoid, e.g. Pigmanorm®. A Cochrane SR identified superiority of triple combination creams over hydroquinone alone. In a study of 641, 26% achieved complete clearance after <u>twice daily application for 8 weeks.</u>
- **Other topicals – in decreasing order of recommendation:** hydroquinone alone (for mild–moderate melasma), azelaic acid (as effective as 4% hydroquinone), topical retinoids.

Step 2

- **Oral tranexamic acid (TA)** [3]: <u>250mg BD for 3 months. Can give repeated courses for recurrence.</u> History should screen for thrombotic risk factors, otherwise no blood tests are necessary unless strong clinical concern. A placebo-controlled RCT of 39 patients found a 49% reduction in MASI score in the TA group vs 18% in the control group.

Step 3

- **Chemical peels** [4]: glycolic acid peels are most widely used. But recurrence is common, and the risk of pigmentary change, particularly in darker skin types, is a noteworthy concern.
- **Lasers (e.g. non-ablative fractional, QS-Nd:YAG, PDL)** [4]: recurrence is common. Intermittent treatment may be required.

Handbook of Skin Disease Management, First Edition. Zainab Jiyad and Carsten Flohr.
© 2023 John Wiley & Sons Ltd. Published 2023 by John Wiley & Sons Ltd.
Companion website: www.wiley.com/go/jiyad/handbookofskindiseasemanagement

Clinical Pearls

- The best results are likely achieved with a combination of different treatments.
- A hormonal factor is implicated in the pathogenesis of melasma, and both OCP and HRT are recognised risk factors. A case series of 4 reported melasma spontaneously improving after switching from COCP to a hormonal-IUD. A discussion with the patient about contraception is recommended.

M

Molluscum contagiosum

A detailed discussion about **treating vs no treatment** is essential. Molloscum in children is self-limiting, and it is important to stress this to parents, as well as side effects of treatments that are common. **Consider treatment** if slow spontaneous clearance, symptomatic, or secondary complications (e.g. eczema, anetoderma-like scarring, conjunctivitis if periorbital). Counsel regarding **auto-innoculation** and **likely duration** (6–9 months, up to several years).

Step 1

- **Potassium hydroxide (KOH)** [1]: 5% (e.g. MolluDab®) or 10% (e.g. MolluTinc®). <u>Apply 3 times a week up to once daily, as tolerated, until clearance.</u> A placebo-controlled RCT of 53 showed efficacy for 10% KOH over placebo, with 64% achieving a reduction in number of molluscum lesions.
- **Hydrogen peroxide 1% cream** [4]: brand name Crystacide®. <u>Use 3 times a week–daily for 3–6 weeks.</u> Particularly helpful for facial molluscum.
- **Salicylic acid** [2]: commonly used, in variable strength (higher for acral sites). Variable regimens, as tolerated (<u>e.g. 3 times a week</u>).
- **Podophyllotoxin** [2]: <u>apply paint twice daily for 3 consecutive days, repeat as necessary.</u> In a placebo-controlled RCT of 150, 92% in treatment group resolved vs 16% in placebo group. Also useful in ano-genital disease.

Step 2

- **Cryotherapy** [2]: <u>used weekly</u> found to be superior to imiquimod in one study. Limited to treating small numbers of lesions and side effects (pain, bullae, pigmentary change, scarring).

Refractory

- **Topical retinoids** [2]: a RCT of 50 of topical tretinoin vs 5% KOH found both reduced mean lesion count at 4 weeks, but retinoids were better tolerated.
- **Imiquimod** [3]: although widely used, a Cochrane review concluded there was moderate-quality evidence that imiquimod was no more effective than vehicle. <u>Use as per warts (page 177), 3 times a week.</u>
- **Curettage** [3]: in a prospective study of 73, curettage failed to resolve lesions in 66% at week 4.
- **Cantharidin** [2]: applied by clinician to molluscum with cotton swab, repeated every 2–4 weeks. Evidence of superiority over placebo in a pilot RCT of 94 patients (36% clearance at 6 weeks).
- **Others:** pulsed dye laser, silver nitrate, trichloroacetic acid, electrodessication. **Immunosuppressed patients:** topical cidofovir, imiquimod, or interferon.

Handbook of Skin Disease Management, First Edition. Zainab Jiyad and Carsten Flohr.
© 2023 John Wiley & Sons Ltd. Published 2023 by John Wiley & Sons Ltd.
Companion website: www.wiley.com/go/jiyad/handbookofskindiseasemanagement

Morphoea

The different subtypes of morphoea require specific treatment approaches (*see overleaf*). The goal of treatment is to reduce inflammation, soften areas of sclerosis, and minimise damage, e.g. skin atrophy, soft tissue loss, and joint contractures. The skin may not return to normal appearance. Severity of disease, and thus treatment escalation, depends on **i) disease activity** (*see next page for how to assess this*), **ii) depth of involvement, iii) site and extent of skin involvement,** and **iv) impact of the disease** on the patient. Appropriate investigations are outlined *overleaf.* Extracutaneous symptoms including headache, myalgia, arthralgia and fatigue, dyspnoea, and dysphagia may occur and require symptomatic therapy. A higher prevalence of concurrent and familial autoimmune disease is documented. It is important to consider the psychosocial impact and offer support.

Circumscribed superficial

- **Potent/superpotent TCS** [4]: OD/BD. Best used for inflammatory areas. 6–12-week trial. IL steroids sometimes used at dose of 10mg/mL into affected areas.
- **Topical tacrolimus 0.1%** [4]: BD to affected areas, with or without occlusion. In an uncontrolled study of 13 patients, 7 improved by more than 70%.
- **Vitamin D analogues** [3]: in an open-label study, all 12 patients who applied topical calcipotriene BD under occlusion for 3 months showed a statistically significant improvement. Use BD, with or without occlusion.
- **If above fail consider imiquimod** [4] **> proceed with phototherapy > methotrexate, as below, if appropriate.**

  Deep disease usually requires systemic treatment, as per management for linear/ pansclerotic.

Generalised

- **Phototherapy** [4]: *usually first-line for generalised morphoea.* Although a Cochrane SR identified no differences between UVA1/UVB, UVA1 is preferred for deep disease/ rapidly progressive (if available).
- **Hydroxychloroquine** [3]: consider in extensive superficial disease.
- **Methotrexate +/- steroids** [4]: RCT of 70 children showed superiority of combination of prednisolone for 3 months with MTX. Approximate one-third relapsed vs 71% in those treated with prednisolone alone. Although steroid monotherapy has lost favour, steroids are important adjunctive tx for severe/rapidly progressing disease: use pulsed methylprednisolone (30mg/kg/day for 3 consecutive days of a month) or oral 1mg/kg.

  If these treatments fail, proceed with MMF > others as below.

Handbook of Skin Disease Management, First Edition. Zainab Jiyad and Carsten Flohr.
© 2023 John Wiley & Sons Ltd. Published 2023 by John Wiley & Sons Ltd.
Companion website: www.wiley.com/go/jiyad/handbookofskindiseasemanagement

Morphoea

M

Linear/ Pansclerotic/ deep/ refractory

- **Assess functional impairment.**
- **For limb disease:** if any impairment or *if at risk* of this, refer to physio, OT, orthopaedics, and rheumatology.
- **For head and neck disease:** refer all to ophthalmology. Check for neurological symptoms and dental/jaw involvement and refer to neurology and maxilla-facial surgeons, as appropriate. **Baseline MRI recommended in all head and neck morphoea.**
- **Methotrexate +/- steroids** [4]: *treatment of choice,* as above.
- **MMF** [3]: usually 1g BD. In a retrospective review, 60% of 73 patients showed improvement after 3–6 months.
- **Abatacept:** in severe or unresponsive disease 125mg s/c weekly +/- intravenous induction 0.5–1g at baseline and weeks 2 and 4.
- **Others** [4]: hydroxychloroquine [3], ciclosporin, tocilizumab, tofacitinib, infliximab, rituximab, extracorporeal photopheresis. Fat transfer and fillers may be of value, particularly in head and neck disease.

Circumscribed
- Round to oval plaque(s) >1 cm in diameter, in up to two of seven anatomical regions (head–neck, each limb, anterior trunk, posterior trunk)
- Most common form

Generalised
- Occurrence of multiple plaques of morphoea at three or more anatomical sites in an isomorphic or non-isomorphic distribution
- Most often superficial

Linear
- Linear involvement
- Blashkoid distribution
- Dermis and subcutis (may extend to muscle and bone)
- Most common subtype in children
- 2 main types: trunk & limb variant, head & neck variant including en coup de sabre and Parry-Romberg (also known as progressive hemifacial atrophy).

Pansclerotic
- Circumferential involvement of the majority of body surface areas with sparing of fingers, toes and nipples.
- Affects the dermis and frequently the subcutis, fascia, muscle and/or bone.
- Can be difficult to distinguish from systemic sclerosis but has negative SSc-Specific ANA and normal nailfold capillaroscopy.
- Significant morbidity
- Risk of SCC in children

Mixed
- Combination of 2 or more of other subtypes.

All forms of morphoea can be superficial or deep.

Which investigations to request?

- Diagnosis is usually clinical, but a **skin biopsy** can be done if the diagnosis is in doubt, or to ascertain depth of involvement. It should be a deep incisional ellipse extending through the edge and to the subcutis.
- **ANA** is positive in 5.9–68% of morphoea patients. Factors that have been identified as predictive of relapse in morphoea include ANA positivity, older age of diagnosis, and longer delay in treatment.
- **Other autoantibodies** do not have clear prognostic value, and routine testing is not recommended at present.
- Serological testing for **Borrelia burgdorferi** may be indicated in selected cases where hx is suggestive.
- If involvement beyond dermis or fasciitis is suspected, or if linear head and neck disease, **MRI** should be performed. It has benefit in assessing depth of involvement and monitoring response to treatment.

How to assess disease activity?

This can be notoriously difficult.

- **History:** extension of existing or new lesions.
- **Examination:** erythema, oedema, expansion, and induration are signs of activity. Inactive lesions tend to be atrophic and hyperpigmented.
- **Photography:** helps track changes.
- **Scoring:** the Localized Scleroderma Assessment Tool (LoSCAT) is a validated tool.
- **Other techniques:** MRI, ultrasound, infrared thermography and durometry all have proven use in monitoring, with appropriate clinical correlation.

Mycosis fungoides (MF)

Management below pertains to **early stage MF** (*stages IA–IIA; see overleaf for grading*). More advanced stages or refractory skin disease should be managed in specialist centres. In selected patients with IA, IB, and IIA disease, 'watch and wait' is a reasonable strategy.

All Patients

1) **Skin biopsy:** multiple biopsies often required before diagnosis is made. T-cell gene rearrangement on lesional skin, if available.
2) **Clinical examination: determine lesion type and body surface area (mSWAT),** check lymphadenopathy, organomegaly.
3) **Bloods – some do not advocate testing in IA disease:** FBC, U/Es, LFTs, LDH. Consider HIV and HTLV1 in some cases.
4) **Extended investigations only if hx/examination suggestive:** PET/CT, lymph node biopsy, T-cell subsets, and clonality.

Step 1

- **Potent/superpotent TCS** [3]: <u>OD/BD.</u> In a retrospective study of 200 patients, a 90% response rate was reported.

Step 2

- **Phototherapy** [3]: generally NBUVB used for patch disease and PUVA used for plaques/thicker/resistant areas. Meta-analysis found complete response in 156 of 251 (62%) patients treated with NBUVB vs 389 of 527 (74%) treated with PUVA.
- **Localised radiotherapy** [2]: in a retrospective review, a complete response was seen in 94% of lesions treated with a single fraction of 7–8 Gy.

Step 3

- **Topical nitrogen mustard (mechlorethamine hydrochloride)** [4]: gel (Ledaga®) applied to affected areas <u>once daily.</u> In RCT of 260, ~60% using gel responded (based on severity index). Side effects such as burning are common, consider using with TCS. Small increased risk of keratinocyte cancers, especially with phototherapy.
- **Topical bexoretene** [4]: licensed in US but not in Europe. Trials reported overall response rate of 44–63%. <u>Use BD.</u>

Handbook of Skin Disease Management, First Edition. Zainab Jiyad and Carsten Flohr.
© 2023 John Wiley & Sons Ltd. Published 2023 by John Wiley & Sons Ltd.
Companion website: www.wiley.com/go/jiyad/handbookofskindiseasemanagement

> **Refractory**

- **Usually referred to specialist centre.**
- **Retinoids** [4]: bexoretene most commonly used, see UK consensus protocol for initiation guide (see Bibliography [online]).
- **Interferon-alpha** [3]: often used in combination treatments with PUVA/retinoids/skin-directed therapies.
- **Total skin electron beam (TSEB) therapy** [3]: treatment with adjuvant therapies is usual after TSEB.
- **Methotrexate** [3]: in a study of 29, the response rate was 58%. Often combined with other therapies.
- **Topicals rarely used:** carmustine (BCNU) is not available in the UK, imiquimod.

TNMB staging for MF and Sezary syndrome

Skin (T)	T1	Limited patches, papules, and/or plaques (<10% BSA)		T	N	M	B
	T1a	Patches only	IA	1	0	0	0 / 1
	T1b	Plaques ± patches	IB	2	0	0	0 / 1
	T2	Patches, papules, or plaques covering ≥10% BSA	IIA	1 / 2	1 / 2	0	0 / 1
	T2a	Patches only	IIB	3	0-2	0	0 / 1
	T2b	Plaques ± patches	IIIA	4	0-2	0	0
	T3	One or more tumours (≥1cm diameter)	IIIB	4	0-2	0	1
	T4	Confluence of erythema covering ≥80% body surface area	IVA$_1$	1-4	0-2	0	2
			IVA$_2$	1-4	3	0	0-2
Nodes (N)	N0	No clinically abnormal peripheral lymph nodes	IVB	1-4	0-3	1	0-2
	N1	Clinically abnormal peripheral lymph nodes; histopathology Dutch grade 1 or NCI LN$_{0-2}$					
	N1a	Clone negative					
	N1b	Clone positive					
	N2	Clinically abnormal LNs; histopathology Dutch grade 2 or NCI LN$_3$					
	N2a	Clone negative					
	N2b	Clone positive					
	N3	Clinically abnormal peripheral lymph nodes; histopathology Dutch grades 3–4 or NCI LN$_4$					
Visceral (M)	M0	No visceral organ involvement					
	M1	Visceral involvement (must have pathology confirmation and organ involved should be specified)					

Blood (B)	B0		Absence of significant blood involvement (≤5% of peripheral blood lymphocytes are atypical/Sezary cells)
		B0a	Clone negative
		B0b	Clone positive
	B1		>5% of peripheral blood lymphocytes are atypical (Sezary) cells but does not meet the criteria of B2
		B1a	Clone negative
		B1b	Clone positive
	B2		High blood tumour burden defined as one of the following: ≥1000/microL Sezary cells; CD4:CD8 ratio ≥10 with positive clone; or CD4$^+$ CD7$^-$ cells ≥40% or CD4$^+$ CD26$^-$ cells ≥30% with positive clone

Palmoplantar keratoderma (PPK)

Distinction should be made between hereditary and acquired PPK. There are a great many causes for the latter, including drugs, systemic disease, malignancy, and dermatoses. Treating the underlying cause is central to the management of acquired PPK. Genetic testing should be offered for inherited PPK if the family mutation is not known (in the UK, NHS Genomic Medicine Service PPK panel).

All Patients

1) **Recommend using wicking socks** to absorb moisture for patients with hyperhidrosis.
2) **Regular podiatry review** to pare down calluses, though some patients pare down their own calluses.
3) **Insoles/orthotics.**
4) **Good skin care and treat infection, e.g tinea** – the latter can be a cause of worsening pain.

Step 1

- **Keratolytics** [4]: salicylic acid or urea commonly used. Variable concentrations for salicylic acid – can be compounded with propylene glycol in concentrations from 5 to 10% (start lower) and left overnight under occlusion. Various preparations containing urea from 5 to 40% are available.
- **Topical steroids** [4]: occasionally used with other topicals, particularly if symptomatic or inflammatory component.
- **Topical retinoids** [4]: can be combined with oral retinoids and topical steroids.
- **Calcipotriol** [4]: case reports of improvement, in combination with oral retinoids.

Step 2

- **Oral retinoids** [3]: acitretin most widely used (standard dosing, page 191), but in child-bearing women, alitretinoin can be used as an alternative. Isotretinoin may be less efficacious.
- **Botox** [4]: case reports of improvement in calluses, blistering, and symptoms with palmoplantar injections.

Handbook of Skin Disease Management, First Edition. Zainab Jiyad and Carsten Flohr.
© 2023 John Wiley & Sons Ltd. Published 2023 by John Wiley & Sons Ltd.
Companion website: www.wiley.com/go/jiyad/handbookofskindiseasemanagement

Refractory

- **Oral and topical sirolimus** [4]: topical sirolimus in clinical trials for Pachyonychia congenita. In an open study of 3 patients with Pachyonychia congenita, oral sirolimus improved PPK but was stopped due to side effects.
- **Others:** erlotinib (for Olmsted syndrome), rosuvastatin (case report), surgery may be required in cases of severe pseduoainhum.

Papular urticaria

This is secondary to insect bites, though often the culprit can be difficult to identify. It should be differentiated from papular eczema and other conditions that may appear similar. Elimination of the cause is a central step in management.

All Patients

1) **Pets** should investigated for fleas by a veterinarian.
2) If bedbugs or fleas are suspected, **fumigation of a property** should be undertaken.
3) **Clothes and bedding** should be washed at high temperatures.
4) **A skin biopsy** can be undertaken to confirm the diagnosis.

Step 1

- **Antihistamines** [2]: use non-sedating antihistamines, e.g. *fexofenadine 180mg BD*. A sedating antihistamine can be used at night, as required, e.g. hydroxyzine.
- **Potent topical steroids** [4]: often give effective symptom control.
- **Topical antipruritics** [4]: can be combined with oral steroids and topical steroids.

Step 2

- **Oral steroids** [4]: short 5–7-day courses (e.g. *prednisolone 30mg OD*) provide effective and rapid relief, though recurrence is common if the underlying cause has not been eradicated.
- **Insect repellents** [4]: various preparations available over the counter. Permethrin can be used for both treatment and as a repellent.

Refractory

- **Immunosuppressants** [4]: methotrexate or ciclosporin can be used in severe cases.
- **Phototherapy** [4].

Handbook of Skin Disease Management, First Edition. Zainab Jiyad and Carsten Flohr.
© 2023 John Wiley & Sons Ltd. Published 2023 by John Wiley & Sons Ltd.
Companion website: www.wiley.com/go/jiyad/handbookofskindiseasemanagement

Pemphigus vulgaris and foliaceous

Although pemphigus foliaceous tends to be a milder disease, severity is highly variable.

All Patients

1) **Take a skin biopsy for histology (lesional skin) and direct IMF (perilesional skin):** see page 218. Consider testing serum for indirect immunofluorescence as well. Routine bloods and systemics initiation bloods usually performed at diagnosis, as well.
2) **Recommend good skin care as follows:** deflate tense blisters with sterile needle and leave blister roof on; wash with antibacterial lotion; regular use of moisturising ointment; non-adhesive dressings.

Step 1

- **Superpotent TCS** [4]: used adjunctively, though evidence lacking.
- **Mouth care** [4]: see page 12, *apthous ulcers, STEP 1 ONLY.*
- **Oral steroids** [1]: prednisolone 1mg/kg/day (range 0.5–2mg), review and increase as necessary. *See overleaf for tapering guide.* Pulsed steroids are sometimes used: 250–1000mg daily for 3–5 days, esp. for severe/resistant disease.
  Steroid-sparing systemic is usually started concurrently with oral steroids:
- **MMF** [1]: see page 188 for dosing.
- **Or azathioprine** [1]: *most commonly used agent.* See page 185 for dosing. A Cochrane review did not conclude superiority over MMF; however, some individual studies have reported this.
- **Or rituximab** [1]: many experts now recommend first-line use of rituximab, which in trials enables 70% of patients to achieve remission off steroids after 6 months. Early use seems to confer greater likelihood of complete remission.

Step 2

- **Rituximab or further cycles if already on this** [1]: various doses have been used, but most commonly 2 infusions of 1g, 2 weeks apart.

Handbook of Skin Disease Management, First Edition. Zainab Jiyad and Carsten Flohr.
© 2023 John Wiley & Sons Ltd. Published 2023 by John Wiley & Sons Ltd.
Companion website: www.wiley.com/go/jiyad/handbookofskindiseasemanagement

Refractory

- **Intravenous immunoglobulin (IVIG)** ④: 1g/kg or 2g/kg – divided over 5 days. A beneficial effect was demonstrated in a placebo-controlled RCT of 61 patients.
- **Cyclophosphamide** ①: uncommonly used due to toxicity. A Cochrane review found a steroid-sparing effect.
- **Immunoadsorption** ④: limited availability. Differs from plasmapheresis. Some evidence to suggest combination with rituximab achieves faster disease control.
- **Dapsone** ③: sometimes added in to work concurrently with other treatments.
- **Not recommended/little evidence to support efficacy:** plasmapheresis, methotrexate.

How to manage oral corticosteroids?

- Review and increase dose if no improvement after 7–10 days.
- Dose can be tapered if no new blisters after 10–14 days and healing of established lesions.
  - Decrease dose slowly until 15mg is reached, then by 2.5mg every week until 5mg. Subsequently decrease by 1mg decrements thereafter or clinic review – weekly/every few days. Remember bone and gastric prophylaxis and DEXA scan requirements. Patients on rituximab can usually be weaned faster.
- If flares during tapering, go back to the last dose (before flare began).
- If flares after steroid course is complete – restart and consider increasing dose of systemic.
- Assess and manage side effects (e.g. osteoporosis).

Pemphigus subtypes and antigens

	Target antigens	Variants
Pemphigus vulgaris	Desmogleins 1 and 3	• Pemphigus vegetans • Pemphigus herpetiformis
Pemphigus foliaceous	Desmoglein 1	• Fogo selvagem • Pemphigus erythematosus
Paraneoplastic pemphigus	Envoplakin, periplakin, Desmogleins 1 and 3, desmoplakin, plectin, epiplakin, BP230, BP180, Desmocollin 1/2/3, α2-macroglobulin-like protein 1	–
IgA pemphigus	Desmocollins 1, 2 and 3; Desmogleins 1 and 3	• Subcorneal pustular dermatosis-type IgA pemphigus • Intraepidermal neutrophilic dermatosis
Drug-induced pemphigus	–	–

Periorificial dermatitis

Obtain a thorough history of topical applications to face, particularly topical steroid use.

Step 1

- **Stop corticosteroids, emollients, and cosmetics** [4]: explain that they may flare initially with cessation of corticosteroids.
- **Topical pimecrolimus 1%** [4]: use BD. In a multicentre RCT of 124 patients, pimecrolimus was found to be superior to placebo.
- **Topical antibiotics** [2]: use erythromycin 2% gel BD or topical metronidazole OD for 8–14 weeks. In a randomised controlled trial of 108 patients of topical metronidazole vs oral tetracycline, the median number of papules in the metronidazole-treated group was reduced to 8% of the initial number, although oral tetracycline was significantly better.

Step 2

- **Oral tetracyclines (contraindicated in children <12 years)** [4]: doxycycline 100mg OD/BD for 8 weeks. Superiority over topical metronidazole shown as above.
- **Oral erythromycin** [4]: alternative to tetracyclines in children. Use 500mg BD for 8 weeks.

Refractory

- **Azelaic acid** [2]: In a study of 10 patients, 20% azelaic acid used BD until resolution resulted in complete resolution in all children after 4–8 months.
- **Topical ivermectin** [2]: applied once daily for 3 months. A retrospective review showed that 4 children were clear/nearly clear following treatment.
- **Case reports** [4]: adapalene, oral isotretinoin, and oral metronidazole.

Handbook of Skin Disease Management, First Edition. Zainab Jiyad and Carsten Flohr.
© 2023 John Wiley & Sons Ltd. Published 2023 by John Wiley & Sons Ltd.
Companion website: www.wiley.com/go/jiyad/handbookofskindiseasemanagement

Pigmented purpuric dermatoses (PPD)

History should screen for possible drug causes, which include acetaminophen, aspirin, chlordiazepoxide, thiamine, hydralazine, although often no cause is ever identified. The evidence-base for treatment recommendations is largely derived from case series/reports. Subtypes of PPD:

- Eczematoid-like purpura of Doucas and Kapetankis
- Granulomatous variant
- Itching purpura of Loewenthal
- Lichen aureus
- Linear PPD
- Pigmented purpuric lichenoid dermatosis of Gougerot and Blum
- Purpura annularis telangiectaticum (Majocchi's)
- Schamberg's disease
- Transitory PPD

Step 1

- **Compression stockings** [4].
- **Topical corticosteroids** [4]: variable potencies used. Trial potent TCS OD for 6 weeks.
- **Topical calcineurin inhibitors** [4]: some case reports of success. Trial OD/BD for 12 weeks.

Step 2

- **Ascorbic acid and bioflabonoids** [3]: the two are usually combined. In a retrospective review of 35 treated, 71% completely cleared with mean treatment duration of 8.2 months. Use rutoside 50mg BD and ascorbic acid 500mg BD.
- **Phototherapy** [3]: high reports of success (>75%) with both PUVA and NBUVB.

Step 3

- **Colchicine** [4]: Use 500 micrograms start at OD and increase to BD after 1 week, trial for 3 months.
- **Laser/intense pulsed light (IPL) therapy** [4]: case reports of success with IPL as well as various lasers, including alexandrite and erbium:glass.

Handbook of Skin Disease Management, First Edition. Zainab Jiyad and Carsten Flohr.
© 2023 John Wiley & Sons Ltd. Published 2023 by John Wiley & Sons Ltd.
Companion website: www.wiley.com/go/jiyad/handbookofskindiseasemanagement

Refractory

- **Pentoxifylline** ②: use 400mg BD for 3 months. In a study of 112, 61% improved, compared with 21% in TCS group.
- **Ciclosporin** ④: should only be considered as a last resort, where appropriate. Standard dosing, see page 183.
- **Other:** griseofulvin – an open trial of 6 reported improvement in 5 patients using 500–750mg OD within 7–10 days. Though no reasonable mechanism for effectiveness, so results unlikely to be reproducible.

Pityriasis lichenoides

Pityriasis lichenoides et varioliformis acuta **(PLEVA)** and pityriasis lichenoides chronica **(PLC)** are thought to exist on a spectrum, and treatment here pertains to both, although frequently a conservative approach is taken with PLEVA, which is usually self-limiting. Note, the *duration of PLEVA is highly variable* – a retrospective study of 71 children found a median duration of PLEVA of 18 months (range 4–108 months), and the condition may relapse and remit over this period.

Step 1

- **Potent TCS** [3]: although frequently used, evidence is based on uncontrolled studies. A recent SR reported that in isolation, TCS were associated with complete response in only 4% of patients (2/45) and a partial response in 80% (20/25). Patients symptomatic with itch often find relief. Trial for 6 weeks.

Step 2

- **Tetracyclines** [3]: usually doxycycline 100mg BD, for 6–12 weeks. In a SR of 17 included patients, a complete response was reported in 53% and a partial response in 35%. **Do not use in children.**
- **Erythromycin** [3]: use in children. 30–50mg/kg/day for 6–12 weeks. In a study of 57 with PLC or PLEVA who were treated with erythromycin, 67% improved in ~2 months.
- **Phototherapy** [3]: typically NBUVB is used. In a study of 25, more than 90% had at least partial improvement (50%+). In a SR, of 136 patients, 102 (75%) achieved a complete response. A typical regime is 3 times a week for 3 months, tapered as appropriate PUVA, UVA1, and BBUVB have also been used.

Refractory

- **Methotrexate** [4]: in a case series of 6, all were reported to achieve a complete response. Standard dosing (see page 181).
- **Others, case reports** [4]: topical tacrolimus, dapsone, retinoids, ciclosporin, IVIG.

Handbook of Skin Disease Management, First Edition. Zainab Jiyad and Carsten Flohr.
© 2023 John Wiley & Sons Ltd. Published 2023 by John Wiley & Sons Ltd.
Companion website: www.wiley.com/go/jiyad/handbookofskindiseasemanagement

Pityriasis rubra pilaris (PRP)

Determining the subtype enables prognostication.

Type	Nomenclature	Characteristic
I	Classical adult	Commonest type (55% of cases), cephalocaudal progression, 'suberythroderma' with islands of sparing and palmoplantar keratoderma.
II	Atypical adult	Ichthyosiform dermatitis, coarse palmoplantar keratosis, sparse scalp hair. Protracted course.
III	Classic juvenile	Similar to type I PRP affects children in the first decade, frequent spontaneous resolution.
IV	Circumscribed juvenile	Sharply demarcated erythema and follicular hyperkeratosis predominantly on the knees and elbows, no progression, course rather protracted.
V	Atypical juvenile	Early onset (first years of life) and chronic course. Follicular hyperkeratosis and ichthyosiform dermatitis.
VI	HIV-related	Nodulocystic and lichen spinulosus-like lesions. Erythroderma as a frequent complication.

Source: Roenneberg S, Biedermann T. Pityriasis rubra pilaris: algorithms for diagnosis and treatment. J Eur Acad Dermatology Venereol 2018;32(6):889–98.

Step 1

- **Medium potency/potent TCS** [3]: topicals best for limited disease/paediatric patients, otherwise use adjunctively.
- **Topical retinoids** [4]: for limited disease, e.g. type IV. Use with TCS can reduce irritation.
- **Emollients +/- urea +/- salicylic acid** [4]: keratolytics are particularly useful for keratoderma.

Step 2

- **Oral retinoids** [4]: isotretinoin preferred, *dose of 0.5–1mg/kg/day, though some use doses of 2mg/kg/day*. Acitretin and alitretinoin are alternatives. In a SR, 102/167 (61%) treated with isotretinoin improved.
- **Methotrexate** [3]: *standard dosing, see page 181*. SR of 116 reported overall response rate of 65.5% with complete clearing in 23.3% and excellent improvement in 17.2%.
- **Phototherapy** [3]: both NBUVB and PUVA used, though efficacy is thought to be poor (1 of 13 in retrospective review). Has been used adjunctively with retinoids.

Refractory

- **Ciclosporin or azathioprine** ④: success reported in case series.
- **Biologics** ③: most evidence based on reports of infliximab use (+/- retinoid), but most biologics (incl. IL17, IL23) have shown success in treating refractory PRP. Some advocate use first-line where disease is extensive or severe.
- **Others:** apremilast, calcipotriol, IVIG, fumaric acid esters, MMF.

Pityriasis versicolor

It is important to explain to patients that pigment change can persist for months after the resolution of infection and that recurrence is common.

Clinical Pearl

Under Wood's lamp PV fluoresces yellow/green/gold; however, reports of test positivity are highly varied (30-88%).

A meta-analysis found insufficient evidence to suggest one topical agent over another, but longer durations of treatment and higher concentrations of active agents produce greater cure rates.

Step 1

- **Medicated shampoos** [1]: ketoconazole 2%, selenium sulphide 2.5%, or zinc pyrithione 1 or 2%. Applied on skin as a shower gel and left on for 5–10 mins, then washed. This should be done daily when showering for 1–4 weeks.
- **Topical azoles** [1]: see page 220. Usually 2 weeks of treatment suffices, sometimes 4 weeks required.

Step 2

- **Oral antifungals** [1]: these are rarely used for severe disease. Short courses of 1–2 weeks are sufficient. Commonly used agents are oral itraconazole 200mg OD for 7 days, fluconazole 50mg daily for 2 weeks or 300mg one dose weekly for 2 weeks. Studies examining itraconazole have reported mycological cure rates typically above 70%. Similar cure rates have been reported with fluconazole from trials including RCTs.
  Ketoconazole is NOT recommended due to safety concerns.

Prophylaxis

In patients with recurrent disease, the following are helpful for prophylaxis:

- **Medicated shampoos** [4]: applied as above once or twice a month (frequency can be increased if recurrence occurs).
- **Oral itraconazole** [4]: in a RCT, 90/102 patients treated with itraconazole 200mg BD for only 1 day per month achieved mycological cure at the end of 6 months.

Handbook of Skin Disease Management, First Edition. Zainab Jiyad and Carsten Flohr.
© 2023 John Wiley & Sons Ltd. Published 2023 by John Wiley & Sons Ltd.
Companion website: www.wiley.com/go/jiyad/handbookofskindiseasemanagement

Polyarteritis nodosa (PAN)

The key step in management is differentiating cutaneous PAN from systemic PAN. These are largely considered distinct entities, and cutaneous PAN rarely, if ever, progresses to systemic PAN. Treatment below pertains to management of cutaneous PAN.

All Patients

1) **Focused history** screening for systemic symptoms.
2) **Skin biopsy** should be undertaken – deep enough to determine involvement of medium-sized vessels (i.e. to subcutis).
3) **Ix:** FBC, U/Es, LFTs, ESR, CRP, ANCA, ANA, Complement, hep B + C, ASOT, cryoglobulins, CXR, ECG. Urine dipstick.

Course of oral steroids can be used for acute flares, usually as weaning regimen.

Step 1

- **Elevation +/- compression stockings** [4].
- **Potent TCS** [4]: can help with symptoms of pain, erythema, burning, or itch.
- **NSAIDs** [3]: ibuprofen commonly used, although alternatives work as well. 400mg TDS/QDS, can use maximum dose of 2400mg/day.

Step 2

- **Colchicine** [3]: 500 micrograms start at OD and increase to BD after 1 week, as tolerated, to maximum of 2mg.
- **Dapsone** [3]: see page 186 for initiation, dose, and monitoring.
- **Hydroxychloroquine** [3]: 200mg OD/BD.
- **Methotrexate** [3]: see page 181 for initiation, dose, and monitoring.

Refractory

- **Azathioprine** [3]: see page 185 for initiation, dose, and monitoring.
- **Pentoxifylline** [3]: 400mg BD/TDS.
- **Others:** IVIG, cyclophosphamide, TNF alpha-inhibitors.

Handbook of Skin Disease Management, First Edition. Zainab Jiyad and Carsten Flohr.
© 2023 John Wiley & Sons Ltd. Published 2023 by John Wiley & Sons Ltd.
Companion website: www.wiley.com/go/jiyad/handbookofskindiseasemanagement

Polymorphic light eruption (PLE)

The diagnosis of PLE is typically clinical and largely based on the history. A photosensitivity screen and phototesting are only required if deemed necessary/appropriate, such as in atypical or severe disease, particularly to rule out lupus.

Step 1

- **Photoprotection** [4]: behaviour, hats, clothing, and regular application of high SPF sunscreen should be encouraged, as well as protective clothing.
- **Potent TCS** [4]: can be beneficial for treating the acute eruption.

Step 2

- **Photohardening** [4]: phototherapy given in early spring can help reduce severity of PLE over summer. In a comparative study of 25 patients, PUVA and NBUVB were found to be similarly efficacious. Some patients may also be able to achieve hardening through repeated low-level natural sunlight exposures.
- **Oral steroids** [4]: short 7-day courses are useful for severe eruptions and can be supplied to patients, particularly for those likely to flare whilst going abroad.

Refractory

- **Antimalarials** [4]: in a placebo-controlled RCT, patients treated with hydroxychloroquine during summer months were reported to have a moderate clinical improvement. A further RCT found hydroxychloroquine to be superior to chloroquine. However, in practice antimalarials are of limited use in PLE.
- **Immunosuppressants** [4]: case reports of successful treatment with azathioprine and ciclosporin have been described.

Emerging: consider vitamin D supplementation. Vitamin D levels in 23 patients were compared with 23 sex/age/BMI–post-hoc matched controls. PLE patients were noted to have significantly lower levels that improved with UVB photohardening. Further, an intraindividual study using pre-treatment with vitamin D analogues (calcipotriol) vs placebo found a significant improvement, with calcipotriol reducing the PLE test score.

Handbook of Skin Disease Management, First Edition. Zainab Jiyad and Carsten Flohr.
© 2023 John Wiley & Sons Ltd. Published 2023 by John Wiley & Sons Ltd.
Companion website: www.wiley.com/go/jiyad/handbookofskindiseasemanagement

Porokeratosis

Although rare, there is a risk of malignant transformation (usually SCC) with most subtypes. This risk is highest with linear porokeratosis and porokeratosis of Mibelli. Destructive therapies work best, but use is limited by the number and extent of lesions and scarring.

Different subtypes of porokeratosis may respond to different treatments:

- Disseminated superficial actinic porokeratosis
- Disseminated superficial porokeratosis
- Porokeratosis of Mibelli
- Porokeratosis ptychotropica
- Linear porokeratosis
- Porokeratosis plantaris palmaris et disseminata
- Punctate porokeratosis

Step 1

- **5-FU** [4]: can be used with or without occlusion – e.g. daily for 8 weeks.
- **Topical vitamin D analogues** [4]: e.g. calcipotriol BD for 3 months.
- **Imiquimod** [4]: variable regimens used. Use as tolerated.
- **Topical retinoids** [4]: case reports/series reporting success, e.g. topical tretinoin daily for 3 months.
- **Cryotherapy** [4]: case reports of improvement.
- **Curettage** [4]: best for few lesions.

Step 2

- **Laser treatment** [4]: various lasers used including Er:YAG, Nd:YAG, and CO_2.
- **Systemic retinoids** [4]: acitretin most commonly used – 3–4-month course improved lesions in case reports.
- **PDT** [4]: most case reports/series report poor efficacy.
- **Other:** topical diclofenac, topical steroids, topical tacrolimus, systemic steroids, oral tacrolimus, and electrochemotherapy have all been reported.

Pruritus

Many skin conditions are pruritic. This section relates to generalised pruritus in the absence of a skin disease, with a specific section on *renal pruritus, overleaf.* Guidelines exist for management of other forms of pruritus (hepatic, malignant and others), *see Bibliography (online).*

All Patients

1) **Take a detailed hx screening for secondary causes of pruritus:** drugs, pregnancy, renal disease, malignancy, liver disease, iron-related disorder, heart failure, endocrine disease, haematological disorders.
2) **Focused examination:** check for lymphadenopathy, organomegaly, and signs of secondary causes such as liver disease.
3) **Baseline screening investigations:** FBC, ferritin, U&E, LFT, ESR/CRP, CXR, vitamin D, TFTs.
4) **Consider additional bloods:** blood film, HBA1C, LDH, bone profile, immunoglobulins, vitamin D, HIV, viral hepatitis, antimitochondrial antibodies.

Treatment of idiopathic generalised pruritus:

Step 1

- **Moisturisers** [4]: creams/ointments – can trial several to find one that suits the patient.
- **Menthol** [4]: ointment or cream vehicle, use QDS. 2% in aqueous cream usually available. Placing menthol/moisturisers in the fridge can provide a beneficial cooling effect.
- **TCS** [4]: potent TCS applied to particularly pruritic areas. Use OD/BD. Tacrolimus 0.1% alternative.
- **Topical doxepin** [4]: BD or QDS. Limit use to 2 weeks. There are concerns re: allergic contact dermatitis.
- **Antihistamines** [4]: trial non-sedating for 2 months, e.g. fexofenadine 180mg, up to QDS.

Step 2

- **Phototherapy** [4]: NBUVB, BBUVB, or PUVA. Most evidence based on studies of renal pruritus.

Handbook of Skin Disease Management, First Edition. Zainab Jiyad and Carsten Flohr.
© 2023 John Wiley & Sons Ltd. Published 2023 by John Wiley & Sons Ltd.
Companion website: www.wiley.com/go/jiyad/handbookofskindiseasemanagement

Refractory

Choose agent to match existing comorbidities (e.g. anticonvulsants if pain/mood disturbances, etc.):

- **Antidepressants** [3]: paroxetine (20mg OD)/fluvoxamine/mirtazapine (10–20mg/day).
- **Anticonvulsants** [4]: gabapentin started at 300mg on the first day, then 300mg BD and then increased to 300mg TDS on third day. Gabapentin can be increased up to 600mg 3 times a day over 3–4 weeks if there is no effect. **OR** pregabalin 75mg BD and increased to 150mg BD after 5–8 weeks.
- **Others:** naltrexone (50–100mg/day), butorphanol, ciclosporin.

Treatment of renal pruritus:

Step 1

- **Optimise dialysis:** ensure Kt/V [marker of dialysis adequacy = (dialyser urea clearance × time)/urea distribution volume] of 1.2 [2], biocompatible membrane [2], high-flux dialyser [4].
- **Optimise blood parameters** [2]: target calcium, phosphate, parathyroid hormone, and haemoglobin levels in accordance with Renal Association guidelines, as per renal function.
- **Moisturiser +/- additives** [4]: cream/ointment – can trial several to find one that suits the patient. Additions of menthol/lauromacrogols (e.g. Balneum plus®) can be beneficial.
- **Topical capsaicin** [4]: use QDS to localised areas of severe itch, up to 6 weeks.
- **Topical calcipotriol** [2]: use BD. An open-label trial of 23 patients found a significant reduction in pruritus score and visual analogue scale, compared with vehicle at 2 and 4 weeks.

Step 2

- **NBUVB phototherapy** [2]: an uncontrolled study found that 32 out of 38 patients with uraemic pruritus improved after a course of 6–8 UVB exposures. There is better evidence for BBUVB, although limited availability. Note – it may be difficult for dialysis patients to attend for phototherapy, and so this may not be a practical option.
- **Gabapentin** [3]: a meta-analysis of 4 studies found 82% reduction in pruritus scores compared with placebo (95% CI 0.09–0.33). Start at 100mg after each dialysis session. Increase dose gradually to max of 300mg daily.

> **Refractory**
>
> - **Antihistamines** ②: though frequently used, British Association of Dermatologists guidelines recommend avoidance because of the association with dementia.
> - **Antidepressants:** sertraline ② (25–200mg daily) or mirtazapine ④ (15–30mg daily).
> - **Topical cromlyn sodium** ④: BD use in an RCT of 60 showed benefit compared to placebo.
> - **Naltrexone** ④: 50mg OD. 1 RCT showed benefit, but a subsequent RCT showed no benefit.
> - **Oral activated charcoal** ④: in a cross-over study of 11 patients, 6g daily of tx improved all but 1 patient.
> - **Montelukast** ④: 10mg OD in 16 patients in 1 RCT showed benefit compared with placebo.
> - **Others:** thalidomide ④ (100mg at night), pregabalin ④ (start at 25mg daily and increase gradually to 75mg daily).

Pseudofolliculitis barbae

Although discontinuation of shaving/other hair removal resolves the condition in a few weeks (up to a few months), this is not a feasible option for many.

Preventative care:
• Pre-shave regimen with warm water and antibacterial soap.   • Key is to avoid a close shave, and use of electric clippers leaving a minimum hair length of 1mm is highly recommended.   • Avoiding pulling skin taught during shave.   • Shave in the direction of hair growth, not against it.   • Rinse the blade with warm water after each shave stroke.   • After care: cool compresses and aftershave cream/lotion.

Step 1

- **Preventative measures:** as outlined above.
- **Chemical depilatories** [4]: come in various preparations, including creams, lotions, and powders. Alternative to shaving.
- **Moderate potency TCS** [4]: provide effective relief of active lesions.
- **Topical retinoids** [3]: use in combination with TCS, some benefit shown in uncontrolled studies.
- **Topical antimicrobials** [2]: mostly used adjunctively, e.g. topical clindamycin. In a pilot placebo-controlled RCT, the use of antimicrobials reduced lesion counts significantly up to 6 weeks, but this was not sustained at 10 weeks.

Step 2

- **Tetracyclines** [4]: course of tetracyclines, similar to use in acne, e.g. *lymecycline 408mg OD for 3 months* may provide relief in some cases.

Refractory

- **Laser hair removal** [2]: various lasers have been used including Nd:YAG and alexandrite, with significant improvements reported.
- **Others:** electrolysis, topical eflornithine, chemical peels.

Handbook of Skin Disease Management, First Edition. Zainab Jiyad and Carsten Flohr.
© 2023 John Wiley & Sons Ltd. Published 2023 by John Wiley & Sons Ltd.
Companion website: www.wiley.com/go/jiyad/handbookofskindiseasemanagement

Psoriasis

Treatment below pertains to chronic plaque psoriasis, but particular subtypes require different approaches – listed on next page. Disease extent and severity determine the initiating treatment, e.g. for widespread disease (>10% BSA), treatment beyond topicals would usually be the starting point.

All Patients

1) **Screen for metabolic syndrome and reduce cardiovascular risk,** where possible with lifestyle and behaviour modifications.
2) Assess impact on **quality of life, perform DLQI, and screen for depression.** Refer to psychologist, where needed.
3) **Complete PASI score (NAPSI for nail disease).**
4) Screen for **psoriatic arthritis** (e.g. PEST score).

Step 1

- **Combination TCS/vitamin D analogues** [3]: e.g. Dovobet®, Enstilar foam® OD/BD. TCS potency based on site involved. Combination preparations are easier to apply and popular, though many prescribed individual treatments.
- **Site-specific topical treatments:** see overleaf.

Step 2

- **Phototherapy** [3]: NBUVB most commonly used and preferred. A Cochrane review that compared NBUVB with PUVA found inconsistent results from included studies. PUVA is best for palmoplantar pustulosis.

Step 3

- **Methotrexate** [3]: systemic of choice. *See page 181 for dosing.* Switch to subcutaneous form if limited efficacy with oral treatment. PASI-75 response rate varies from 25 to 90% depending on studies and dose.
- **Ciclosporin** [3]: systemic of choice for rapid control, palmoplantar pustulosis, or those considering conception. *See page 183 for dosing.* PASI-75 response rate varies from 30 to 90% depending on dose.
- **Acitretin** [1]: where above systemics contraindicated, or for pustular psoriasis. Less efficacious than above.

Handbook of Skin Disease Management, First Edition. Zainab Jiyad and Carsten Flohr.
© 2023 John Wiley & Sons Ltd. Published 2023 by John Wiley & Sons Ltd.
Companion website: www.wiley.com/go/jiyad/handbookofskindiseasemanagement

Refractory

- **Biologics** ①: drug choice depends on patient circumstances, comorbidities, and if there is concurrent psoriatic arthritis. *See Appendix B for table to guide choice and dosing.* UK guidelines recommend PASI ≥10 and DLQI >10 and failure of both MTX and CsA (or not tolerated or contraindicated), prior to biologics initiation.
- **Others:** apremilast, fumaric acid esters.

Nail psoriasis

- **Trial topical steroids and topical Vit D analogues.**
- **IL steroids:** can be quite effective. Repeated injections and pain are limiting factors.
- **Ciclosporin:** in a retrospective study, this was found to be the most effective non-biologic for nail disease.
- **Acitretin:** 40% reduction in NAPSI score in retrospective series.
- **PUVA:** 51% reduction in NAPSI score, same study.
- **Methotrexate:** less efficacy than above systemics.
- **Biologics:** most evidence from TNF α-inhibitors but most biologics will also improve nail disease.

Psoriasis in children:

- Evidence is much more limited in this population.
- Similar principles apply – treat severity.
- Awareness of psychosocial impact in school.
- Judicious use of TCS.
- Severe psoriasis in children is uncommon. Phototherapy is often used second-line before systemics.
- Biologics are approved for the treatment of psoriasis in children.

Scalp disease

- **Trial topical steroid scalp application alone first and add vitamin D scalp application if required:** *see page 219.* Start with potent TCS and escalate potency as necessary.
- **Use of keratolytic shampoos with coal tar:** useful as adjunctive treatment particularly for hyperkeratotic disease, e.g. Sebco®, Cocois®, Capasal®.
- **Escalate treatment thereafter as per psoriasis ladder overleaf:** UV combs may be used for scalp disease but limited use. Often systemics are preferred. Biologics can be considered for severe psychosocially disabling disease.

Palmoplantar pustulosis (PPP)

- **Superpotent TCS:** sometimes compounded (propylene glycol, Dermovate, salicylic acid).
- **Topical vitamin D analogues:** use with TCS.
- **PUVA:** better efficacy than NBUVB. Approximately half will have complete or partial response.
- **Acitretin:** first-line systemic for PPP. *See page 191 for dosing.*
- **Methotrexate:** second-line for PPP, unless arthritis present.
- **Other systemics (ciclosporin)/biologics:** escalate as per treatment ladder overleaf.

Flexural psoriasis

- **Mild–moderate potency TCS:** avoid higher strengths.
- **Vitamin D analogues:** often with TCS.
- **Tacrolimus/pimecrolimus:** effective for facial and intertriginous psoriasis.

Psychodermatology

Psychodermatology is either primary psychiatric disease presenting to dermatology healthcare practitioners (see below) or skin disease in which there are psychological comorbidities. Psychodermatological conditions can be challenging to manage. Treatment via a multidisciplinary team is likely to achieve better outcomes, especially where there is severe disease. Direct confrontation with the patient will seldom result in a positive result and will usually have a detrimental effect on tx.

Body dysmorphic disorder

- The Body Dysmorphic Disorder Questionnaire is a useful and validated screening tool.
- CBT is effective in meta-analysis of RCTs.
- SSRIs are also effective as first-line treatment, based on meta-analysis of RCTs, *e.g. fluoxetine (start 20mg OD, max 60mg OD)*. Higher doses are usually necessary.
- Combination of above may reduce recurrence.
- Second-line = antipsychotic. Best managed by specialist.

Neurotic excoriations

- Psychological interventions: CBT or habit-reversal therapy; both have shown efficacy in studies.
- SSRIs are alternative first-line treatment, *e.g. fluoxetine (start 20mg OD, max 60mg OD)*.
- Case reports of naltrexone benefit.
- Lamotrigine or duloxetine may have some benefit.
- Refer to specialists for further input/support.

Dermatitis artefacta

- Exclude organic disease.
- Usually do not confront.
- Try to establish why the patient is presenting rather than how they are creating the artefact.
- Check for and report any abuse (especially if children).
- Treat skin appropriate to the dermatological presentation.
- Manage in a multidisciplinary team.
- May include dermatitis neglecta and other variations.
- CBT and SSRIs can be initiated by the dermatologist.

Delusions of parasitosis

- Morgellons is a subtype/related disorder where patients believe inanimate objects such as fibres are in the lesions.
- Performing a pruritus screening panel may help to exclude secondary causes of itch and develop rapport.
- Always take seriously and examine the material that patients bring with them (specimen sign).
- Consider recreational drugs/iatrogenic (e.g. opiates) causes.
- Antipsychotics form the mainstay of tx, usually via a psychoderm MDT, *e.g. risperidone, olanzapine.*

Pyoderma gangrenosum

Identification and treatment of an underlying cause is important, particularly in refractory cases.

All Patients

1) **Focused history and examination to identify secondary causes** – see overleaf for list of associations.
2) **Investigations:** see overleaf.
3) **Good wound care is key** – involve specialist nurse.
4) **Pain management.**

Step 1

Topical treatment alone is only appropriate for mild disease, otherwise oral steroids (alternatively CsA) are usually started at the outset, as PG can be both disfiguring and severe:

- **Superpotent TCS** [3]: use OD/BD. In a prospective study, 28 of 66 ulcers (43.8%) treated with topical therapy alone (74.2% TCS, remainder tacrolimus 0.03%) healed by 6 months. Some reports of IL steroid use – caution pathergy.
- **Topical tacrolimus 0.03–0.1%** [3]: OD/BD. Although TCS are preferred treatment, some evidence for tacrolimus: in a study of peristomal PG, 7 of 11 treated with tacrolimus healed completely.
- **Oral steroids** [4]: in a RCT of 112 patients of prednisolone vs ciclosporin for PG, 47% of patients treated in both groups healed. Initiate at 0.5–1mg/kg.
- **Ciclosporin** [4]: as above, similarly efficacious to oral steroids. Start at dose of 4mg/kg, see page 183.

Refractory

- **Biologics** [4]: especially useful in patients with IBD. Infliximab most widely used and studied. In a placebo-controlled trial of 30, 46% in tx arm (5mg/kg every 2 weeks) improved after 2 weeks, vs 6% in placebo arm. Some evidence for other biologics, e.g. adalimumab (variable regimens used). Etanercept is thought to be less efficacious. Based on case reports ustekinumab (17 reports), giselkumab, secukinumab, brodalumab.
- **MMF** [3]: in a retrospective review, 4 of 7 ulcers treated with MMF completely healed. Standard dosing, see page 188.
- **Methotrexate** [4]: based on case reports. Standard dosing, see page 181.
- **Others** [4]: azathioprine, dapsone [3], tetracyclines, colchicine, cyclophosphamide [3], chlorambucil, IVIG [3], thalidomide, alpha interferon, tofacitinib, plasmapheresis, clofazimine.

PG syndromes (e.g. PAPA, PAPASH) respond well to IL-1 antagonists (Anakinra).

Handbook of Skin Disease Management, First Edition. Zainab Jiyad and Carsten Flohr.
© 2023 John Wiley & Sons Ltd. Published 2023 by John Wiley & Sons Ltd.
Companion website: www.wiley.com/go/jiyad/handbookofskindiseasemanagement

Screening investigations for PG

All patients:
- Biopsy from wound edge.
- FBC (+/- blood film) and baseline renal and liver profile.
- Fecal calprotectin in most patients.
- Ensure up-to-date with malignancy screening.

If hx suggestive:
- Endoscopy for IBD.
- Rheumatoid factor and anti-CCP for arthritis +/- imaging.
- ANA and ANCA for connective tissue/vasculitis.
- Further investigation for Behcet's (page 20).
- Appropriate malignancy Ix as per hx.
- Haematology investigations (see below) +/- referral.

If aged ≥ 65:
- Detailed hx and examination for malignancy.
- Blood film.
- Serum and urine electrophoresis.
- Consider referral to haematology.

PG associations

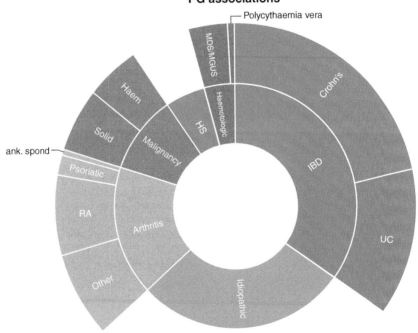

Based on study of 356 confirmed PG cases
Aschyan et al. JAMA Dermatology 2018

Rosacea

There is general consensus that the tx of rosacea should be **phenotype-based**, rather than the subtype, as these can differ and there is overlap between the subtypes (erythematotelangiectatic, papulopustular, phymatous, and ocular). Multiple phenotypes may necessitate a combination of treatments. It is important to identify which features are most troublesome for the patient, to help guide therapeutics. Inflammatory rosacea should be treated first before pursuing procedural therapies.

All Patients

1) **Take a history screening for triggers and recommend avoidance of these:** alcohol, spicy food, exercise, sunlight, etc.
2) **Recommend sun protection:** SPF30+.
3) **Sensitive skin care:** avoid irritants; regular moisturisation and gentle cleansing.

Erythema, flushing, telangiectasia

- **Lasers and intense pulsed light (IPL)** [1]: pulsed dye lasers (PDLs) and IPL most frequently used but KTP lasers have also been trialled. A split-face RCT of 29 patients found similar efficacy for PDL and IPL.
- **Topical alpha-adrenergic receptor agonists** [1]: can be used for persistent erythema. Topical brimonidine gel OD or topical oxymetazoline OD. *There is a risk of rebound erythema, particularly with the former, and some may find worsening of symptoms.* A SR found a reduction in erythema in 41% in the brimonidine group vs 20% of the patients in placebo group. The reduction in erythema was achieved by 22% of the oxymetazoline group vs 13.4% in the placebo group.
- **Oral beta-blockers/α_2-adrenergic agonists** [4]: there is very limited evidence for efficacy in flushing. Use clonidine 50 micrograms BD for 2 weeks, increased to 75 micrograms BD as needed thereafter. Or propranolol 20–40mg BD/TDS.

Handbook of Skin Disease Management, First Edition. Zainab Jiyad and Carsten Flohr.
© 2023 John Wiley & Sons Ltd. Published 2023 by John Wiley & Sons Ltd.
Companion website: www.wiley.com/go/jiyad/handbookofskindiseasemanagement

Inflammatory papules and pustules

MILD:
- **Azelaic acid** [1]: 15% foam/gel or 20% cream/lotion, use BD.
- **Topical ivermectin** [1]: use OD. RCT of 962 found ivermectin more effective vs topical metronidazole.
- **Topical metronidazole** [1]: use 0.75% cream/lotion/gel BD or 1% cream/gel OD.
- **Other topicals – less commonly used:** SR showed poor efficacy for benzoyl peroxide and retinoids.

MODERATE – combine with topicals above:
- **Tetracyclines** [1]: doxycycline 40mg MR/100mg OD or BD/tetracycline 500mg BD/ minocycline 100mg OD or BD. No evidence to suggest minocycline better, and this has more side effects.

SEVERE:
- **Isotretinoin** [4]: in a placebo-controlled RCT of 156, 57% of tx group achieved 90%+ reduction in papules/pustules vs 10% placebo.

Phymatous

Treat inflamed phymatous rosacea first with tetracyclines/isotretinoin before embarking on procedural therapies.
- **Tetracyclines** [1]: doxycycline 40mg MR/100mg OD or BD/tetracycline 500mg BD/ minocycline 100mg OD or BD. Continue for 3–4 months to assess efficacy.
- **Isotretinoin** [4]: limited evidence for improvement in phymatous rosacea. Typically lower doses than those used with acne (0.2–1mg/kg).
- **Surgery/laser treatments:** various methods used including CO_2 lasers, surgical excision, and cryosurgery.

Ocular

- **All but very mild cases are managed by ophthalmologists.**
- **Lid hygiene and artificial tears:** can be prescribed to help with symptoms, pending ophthalmology review.
- **Omega-3 fatty acids through diet or supplements are recommended.**

Sarcoidosis

More than 90% of patients will develop lung disease, refer all to respiratory to co-manage treatment. The treatment algorithm below pertains to cutaneous sarcoidosis. Half of all patients require systemic treatments. Systemic disease may require a more aggressive approach, **including oral steroids (0.5–1mg/kg) if widespread/severe/rapidly progressive.**

All Patients

1) **Focused history screening for systemic disease:** refer to other specialties as indicated, refer all to ophthalmology.
2) **Necessary investigations:** FBC, U/E, LFTs, calcium, ACE level, IL-2, vitamin D (check both 25OH and 1,25OH), TB testing, urine dip, ECG, CXR, lung function tests, skin biopsy. Further tests guided by history and examination.
3) **Most experts recommend baseline:** HRCT, echocardiogram.

Step 1

- **Potent/superpotent TCS** [3]: use OD/BD. Use for active disease only. IL steroids typically used for areas resistant to TCS. Usually 2.5–5mg/mL used.
- **Tacrolimus 0.1% ointment** [4]: likely less efficacious than TCS.

Step 2

- **Hydroxychloroquine** [3]: 200mg OD or BD (max 5mg/kg). In an open trial of 17, 12 had complete response and 3 had partial response, within 12 weeks of treatment. Chloroquine less commonly used.
- **Tetracyclines** [3]: minocycline (100mg BD), alternatively doxycycline can be used (100mg BD). In open study of 12, 8 had complete response to minocycline, 2 partial response. *Can be combined with hydroxychloroquine.*

Step 3

- **Methotrexate** [3]: see page 181 for dosing. A review of studies reported a response rate >80%.

Handbook of Skin Disease Management, First Edition. Zainab Jiyad and Carsten Flohr.
© 2023 John Wiley & Sons Ltd. Published 2023 by John Wiley & Sons Ltd.
Companion website: www.wiley.com/go/jiyad/handbookofskindiseasemanagement

Refractory

- **Thalidomide** [4]: RCT of 39 found no superiority over placebo, after 3 months of tx. But some evidence of efficacy from retrospective series. <u>100–200mg/day</u>. Note lenalidomide is a safer analogue (though no trials).
- **Biologics** [4]: In an observational study of 46 treated with infliximab, the overall cutaneous response rate was 24% after 3 months, 46% after 6 months, and 79% after 12 months. In a RCT of 16 patients of adalimumab vs placebo, a significant improvement in cutaneous sarcoidosis was noted in tx group.
- **Others** [4]: MMF, azathioprine, isotretinoin, allopurinol, tofacitinib, apremilast [3], leflunomide, anti-TB combination drugs [4], UVA1, PUVA, UVB, PDT, lasers.

Scabies

Treatment is directed by subtype – classic vs crusted scabies, and patient age – children vs adults.

All Patients

1) **Cohabitants** also need to be treated at the same time.
2) **Bed linen, clothing, and other items** in contact with skin need to be washed in hot water or kept in a plastic bag for 3 days (scabies mites can survive off the body for 3 days).
3) **Institutions** (e.g. care homes) must be informed to contain the spread of infection.

Step 1

- **Permethrin** [1]: in adults this is applied from the neck downwards. In infants the scalp and face are also included. *This is left on the skin (usually overnight) for 8–14 hrs and then washed off. A second application is applied 1 week later.* A network meta-analysis concluded superiority over other topicals including sulphur and malathion. Malathion can be considered as alternative if permethrin not available.
- **Topical sulphur** [3]: this is sometimes used for very young infants (<3 months) and in pregnant women, though it is less efficacious than permethrin and difficult to obtain.

Step 2

- **Oral ivermectin** [3]: used off-license. For crusted scabies – this is first-line treatment and is used in combination with permethrin. For classic scabies, use *200 micrograms/ kg single dose and repeat 1–2 weeks later.* For crusted scabies, it is *recommended to use the same dose for 3, 5, or 7 non-consecutive days in a 3–4-week period, depending on severity of disease. Permethrin should also be applied every 2–3 days for 1–2 weeks.*

Other

- **Topical spinosad 0.9%** [2]: only recently approved by the FDA, not yet available in UK. No studies to determine efficacy compared with permethrin.
- **Rarely used:** crotamiton, benzyl benzoate, topical ivermectin, monosulphiram.

Handbook of Skin Disease Management, First Edition. Zainab Jiyad and Carsten Flohr.
© 2023 John Wiley & Sons Ltd. Published 2023 by John Wiley & Sons Ltd.
Companion website: www.wiley.com/go/jiyad/handbookofskindiseasemanagement

Scabetic nodules:
Nodules can persist after scabies has been treated. Trial TCS to manage these, after ensuring active scabies has been treated.

Post-treatment pruritus:
Itching can persist for up to 6 weeks after scabies has been treated. TCS can be helpful. Important to differentiate this from reinfestation.

Seborrheic dermatitis

Treatment depends on site and affected surface area. For severe or treatment-resistant seborrheic dermatitis, a HIV test is warranted. Explain to patients that this condition is *chronic* and *relapsing* and topical tx should be *reinstated* during flares.

Step 1

The following topical treatments have similar efficacy, as identified in a Cochrane SR. Usually initiate an azole and combine with PRN use of TCS or topical calcineurin inhibitor.

- **Topical azoles** [1]: most evidence for ketoconazole 2% BD. Usually used until clear, about 10–14 days. See page 220. Often combined with TCS (e.g. Daktacort).
- **Ciclopiroxolamine** [1]: is an alternative available in North America.
- **TCS** [1]: use moderate potency for the face, whilst stronger topicals can be used for the body. Use OD/BD.
- **Topical calcineurin inhibitors** [3]: OD/BD. Useful alternative to TCS, particularly in children.
- **Shampoos for scalp disease** [3]: ketoconazole 2%, zinc pyrithione 1% or selenium sulfide 2.5%. After initial tx phase (2–3 times per week), can use once weekly to prevent relapses. These can also be used for beard/moustache areas.

Shampoos can also be used as a shower gel (left on for 3–5 mins) for disease elsewhere.

Step 2

- **Oral itraconazole** [2]: 200mg daily for 7 days. Intermittent therapy can be given if required thereafter (200mg/day for the first 2 days for 2–11 months). A SR found that 59–93% improved. Courses can be repeated.

Refractory

- **Alternative oral 'azole':** fluconazole [4] (50mg OD for 2–4 weeks). Note ketoconazole carries a weighty risk of hepatotoxicity and is now rarely used for the treatment of skin diseases.
- **Terbinafine** [2]: use 250mg/day for 4 or 6 weeks. One study used a pulse regimen of 250mg/day for 12 days each month for 3 months.

Handbook of Skin Disease Management, First Edition. Zainab Jiyad and Carsten Flohr.
© 2023 John Wiley & Sons Ltd. Published 2023 by John Wiley & Sons Ltd.
Companion website: www.wiley.com/go/jiyad/handbookofskindiseasemanagement

Squamous cell carcinoma (SCC)

Risk categories define treatment for SCC, but note that there is no international consensus on these.

SCC management overview

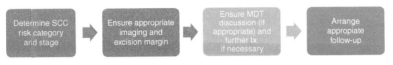

Low risk	High risk	Very high risk
ALL tumor factors below: • Diameter ≤2 mm. • Thickness ≤4 mm. • Invasion into dermis. • No perineural invasion. • Well-differentiated/moderately diffentiated. • No lymphovascular invasion.	**ANY single tumor factor below:** • Diameter 2mm–4mm. • Thickness 4mm–6mm. • Invasion into fat. • Dermal perineural invasion, nerve <0.1mm. • Poorly differentiated. • Lymphovascular invasion. • Tumour on ear/lip. • Tumour within scar or area of chronic inflammation.	**ANY single tumor factor below:** • Diameter >4mm. • Thickness >6mm. • Invasion beyond fat. • Any bone invasion. • Perineural invasion in named nerve; nerve ≥0.1mm, or nerve beyond dermis. • Adenosquamous, desmoplastic, spindle/sarcomatoid/metaplastic. • In-transit metastases.
Clear pathology margins in all directions ≥1mm.	One or more involved/close margin (<1mm) in pT1 tumor, or close margins in pT2 tumor.	One or more involved or close margin in a high-risk tumor.
Immunocompetent.	Immunosuppressed.	Immunosuppressed.

Above: British (BAD) SCC risk categories, **note these differ from widely used NCCN (American, below).**

Handbook of Skin Disease Management, First Edition. Zainab Jiyad and Carsten Flohr.
© 2023 John Wiley & Sons Ltd. Published 2023 by John Wiley & Sons Ltd.
Companion website: www.wiley.com/go/jiyad/handbookofskindiseasemanagement

Below: American (NCCN) SCC risk categories

Low risk	High risk
Area L = trunk/extremities (excluding hands, feet, nail units, pretibia, and ankles) and <20mm OR Area M = cheeks/forehead/scalp/neck/pretibial and <10mm.	Area L ≥20mm. Area M ≥10mm. Any area H = central face, eyelids, eyebrows, periorbital skin, nose, lips, chin, mandible, preauricular and postauricular skin/sulci, temple, ear, genitalia, hands, and feet.
Well-defined borders.	Poorly defined borders.
Primary.	Recurrent.
Immunocompetent.	Immunosuppressed.
NOT site of prior radiation/chronic inflammation.	Site of prior radiation/chronic inflammation.
Not rapidly growing.	Rapidly growing.
No neurological symptoms.	Neurological symptoms.
Well to moderately differentiated.	Poorly differentiated.
No high-risk subtypes.	Adenoid (acantholytic), adenosquamous (showing mucin production), desmoplastic, or metaplastic (carcinosarcomatous) subtypes.
<2mm depth or Clark level I/II/III.	≥2 mm or Clark level IV/V.
No perineural, lymphatic, or vascular involvement.	Perineural, lymphatic, or vascular involvement.

Tables below and above: UICC8 TNM SCC classification and staging, note this differs from AJCC classification.

Primary tumor (T)	Lymph nodes (N) NON- head/neck	Lymph nodes (N) head and neck
T1 ≤2.0cm in greatest dimension	**N1** Metastasis in a single node ≤3cm in greatest dimension	**N1** Metastasis in a single ipsilateral lymph node ≤3cm in greatest dimension without ENE*
T2 >2–4cm in greatest dimension	**N2** Metastasis in a single ipsilateral lymph node, >3cm but ≤6cm or in multiple ipsilateral nodes with none >6cm in greatest dimension	**N2a** Metastasis in a single ipsilateral lymph node >3cm but <6cm in greatest dimension without ENE* **N2b** metastasis in multiple ipsilateral lymph nodes, where none are >6cm in greatest dimension without ENE* **N2c** metastasis in bilateral or contralateral lymph nodes, where none are >6cm in greatest dimension without ENE*
T3 >4cm in greatest dimension or minor bone erosion or perineural invasion (≥0.1mm diameter and/or deeper than the dermis and/or a named nerve) or deep invasion (thickness >6 mm and/or beyond fat)	**N3** metastasis in a lymph node >6cm in greatest dimension	**N3a** metastasis in a single or multiple lymph nodes >6cm in greatest dimension without ENE* **N3b** metastasis in a single or multiple lymph nodes with ENE*
T4a tumour with gross cortical/bone-marrow invasion **T4b** tumour with skull base or axial skeleton invasion		
M category	**M0** no distant metastases	**M1** Distant metastasis (including contralateral nodes in non-head and neck cSCC)

* ENE = extranodal extension.

Stage	T	N	M
I	T1	N0	M0
II	T2	N0	M0
III	T3 T1 / T2 / T3	N0 N1	M0
IVA	T1 / T2 / T3 T4	N2 / N3 Any N	M0
IVB	Any T	Any N	M1

Prognosis:
The overall 5-year survival is generally reported as >95%, with both mortality and metastatic rate reported as <5%.

Acitretin: doses of 10–25mg are commonly prescribed for patients with recurrent SCCs, particularly organ transplant recipients.

Nicotinamide: 500mg BD is also used in patients with recurrent SCCs, especially transplant recipients

Step 2: ensure appropriate imaging and excision margin.

Excision margins UK (BAD)	Excision margins USA (AAD)	Excision margins European (EORTC)
Low risk: ≥4mm	Low risk: 4–6mm	Minimal risk (tumor thickness ≤2mm): 5mm
High risk: ≥6mm	No recommendations on margins for high risk	Low risk (tumor thickness 2.01–6mm): 5–10mm
Very high risk: ≥10mm		High risk (tumor thickness >6mm): 10mm

Imaging?

US local lymph nodes +/- FNA: consider in very-high-risk SCC (BAD), or where there are clinically suspicious nodes.
MRI/CT staging: is undertaken where there is suspicion of metastatic disease/ in transit metastases, or perineural invasion of named nerve.

Step 3: ensure MDT discussion and further treatment (if appropriate).

BAD multidisciplinary meeting recommendations

Low risk: no MDT discussion required.
High risk: local skin cancer MDT discussion if close/involved margins, or more than one factor.
Very high risk: specialist skin cancer MDT discussion.

Radiotherapy?

Primary radiotherapy can be offered where surgery is not feasible.
Adjuvant radiotherapy consider in following:

i) T3 tumor that is completely excised but close (<1mm) margins and multiple high-risk factors, after MDT discussion.
ii) Incompletely excised tumor where further surgery is not feasible and high risk of recurrence (immunosuppressed/perineural invasion/recurrent disease).

Step 4: arrange appropriate follow-up.

UK recommendations (BAD)	USA recommendations (AAD)	European recommendations (EORTC)
Low risk: offer a single appointment to check results, perform skin check, and recommend self-examination	On at least an annual basis	Low risk: every 12 months for 1–5 years
High risk: 4 monthly appointments for 12 months, then 6 monthly for further 12 months		High risk: every 3–4 months for 1–2 years, then every 6 months for years 3–5, then annually after 5th year
Very high risk: 4 monthly appointments for 24 months, then 6 monthly for 12 months		Metastatic disease: every 3 months for 5 years, then annually thereafter
Metastatic disease: 3 monthly appointments for 24 months, then 6 monthly for 36 months with potential long-term review		

Organ transplant recipients should have regular lifelong screening.

Sweet's syndrome

Although in almost half of cases Sweet's is idiopathic, it is important to screen and treat underlying causes.

All Patients

1) **History and examination screening for secondary causes:** URTI, GI infections, TB, HIV, CTDs, IBD, pregnancy, haematological malignancies, solid organ malignancies, G-CSF, minocycline, multiple other medications.
2) **Ix:** FBC, blood film, CRP, U/Es, LFTs, pregnancy test, further screening as directed by history.
3) **Skin biopsy.**

Step 1

- **Oral steroids** [3]: a rapid response to steroids is a key feature of neutrophilic dermatoses, e.g. 30–40mg taper down over 6 weeks.
- **Potent/superpotent TCS** [4]: often used adjunctively.

Step 2

- **Colchicine** [3]: in a retrospective review, 18 of 20 responded to treatment. Use 500 micrograms start at OD and increase to BD after 1 week, as tolerated, to maximum of 2mg.
- **Dapsone** [4]: see page 186 for dosing.

Refractory

- **Potassium iodide** [4]: see page 55 for dosing. Can be difficult to obtain.
- **Ciclosporin** [4]: see page 183 for dosing.
- **Others:** indomethacin, methotrexate, retinoids, thalidomide, anakinra, rituximab, adalimumab.

Handbook of Skin Disease Management, First Edition. Zainab Jiyad and Carsten Flohr.
© 2023 John Wiley & Sons Ltd. Published 2023 by John Wiley & Sons Ltd.
Companion website: www.wiley.com/go/jiyad/handbookofskindiseasemanagement

Telogen effluvium

Differentiate *acute telogen effluvium* (precipitating factor with hair regrowth <12 months) vs *chronic telogen effluvium* (idiopathic, hair loss persists; some have a chronic-repetitive pattern).

All Patients

1) Detailed **history screening** for secondary causes: drugs, recent major illness (e.g. COVID-19), major surgery, childbirth, weight loss, nutritional deficiencies, thyroid disease, inflammatory/infective scalp disorder.
2) **Hair pull test: >6 positive, see page 215.**
3) **Bloods:** FBC, U&Es, LFTs, TFTs, ferritin, folate, B12. Other bloods if there is suggestion of underlying systemic disease, e.g. ANA.
4) **Baseline and follow-up standardised, global photography** to assess response.
5) Recommend **hair camouflage** (see Appendix D)/wigs.

Treatment

- **Treat underlying cause/contributing factors,** if identified. Maintain ferritin levels above 70.
- **Topical minoxidil** [4]: use 5%. Foam preparation has no propylene glycol, which can cause irritation. Treat for at least 4 months before assessing efficacy, hair shedding in first 6 weeks of use can occur. If hair loss resumes on discontinuation, tx should continue indefinitely.
- **Low-dose oral minoxidil (LDOM):** a retrospective review of 36 women identified a mean reduction in the Sinclair shedding scale of 1.7 at 6 and 2.58 at 12 months of treatment with LDOM (dose range 0.25–2.5mg).
- Treat any concurrent **androgenetic alopecia** (see page 57).

Handbook of Skin Disease Management, First Edition. Zainab Jiyad and Carsten Flohr.
© 2023 John Wiley & Sons Ltd. Published 2023 by John Wiley & Sons Ltd.
Companion website: www.wiley.com/go/jiyad/handbookofskindiseasemanagement

Tinea

Scrapings and brushings are essential for confirming the diagnosis and identifying the species.

Tinea corporis/cruris

- **Topical azoles or allyamines** [3]: see page 220. 2 weeks of treatment usually suffices.
- **Oral terbinafine** [4]: for widespread/resistant. 250mg OD 7–10 days.
- **Oral itraconazole** [3]: for widespread/resistant. 200mg OD 7 days.

Tinea pedis

- **Topical allyamines** [1]: see page 220. Marginally more efficacious than azoles. Treat for 4 weeks.
- **Topical azoles** [1]: see page 220. Treat for 4 weeks.
- **Oral terbinafine** [4]: for widespread/resistant. 250mg OD 14 days (fluconazole and griseo fulvin also used).
- **Oral itraconazole** [3]: for widespread/resistant. 200mg OD 7 days.
- **Recurrent cases:** consider use of toe separators, foot powders, treating shoes, non-occlusive footwear, Botox.

Tinea capitis

- **Oral terbinafine** [1]: has emerged as first-line due to shorter courses and greater patient compliance. Higher cure rates for *Trichophyton* infections. Dose dependent on child's weight: 10–20kg=62.5mg daily 4 weeks; 20–40kg=125mg daily for 4 weeks; >40kg=250mg daily for 4 weeks.
- **Griseofulvin** [1]: available as suspension. Best for *Microsporum* infections. 1 month–11 years 10mg/kg/day (max 500mg) increased as required to 20mg/kg/day for 6–12 weeks; 12–17 years: 500mg/day, increased to 1g/day as required, for 6–12 weeks.
- **Itraconazole** [4]: in some countries, this is first-line treatment. Available as suspension. Dose: 3–5mg/kg daily for 2–4 weeks. Pulsed therapy: 3–5mg/kg/day for 1 week each month for 2–3 months.
- **Oral fluconazole** [4]: less commonly used. Dose: 4–6mg/kg for 4–6 weeks. Pulsed therapy: 6mg/kg once weekly for 6–12 weeks.

Handbook of Skin Disease Management, First Edition. Zainab Jiyad and Carsten Flohr.
© 2023 John Wiley & Sons Ltd. Published 2023 by John Wiley & Sons Ltd.
Companion website: www.wiley.com/go/jiyad/handbookofskindiseasemanagement

Tinea capitis clinical pearls

- Adjunctive use of topical shampoos (e.g. ketoconazole) may reduce the carrier state and reduce the spread of infection – most recommend all family members use it.
- Reinfection is not uncommon – family members and pets should be screened.
- Knowing the local species is key: in the UK and USA, *T.tonsurans* is most widespread.
- *M.canis, M.audouinii, M.ferrugineum,* and *M.distorum* fluoresce green-yellow under Wood's lamp.

Tinea unguium (onychomycosis)

- **Topicals (amorolfine, tavoborole, ciclopirox, efinaconazole)** [4]: although poor efficacy, most patients will have tried this prior to dermatological assessment. Applied to nail once daily for 48 weeks. Best combined with oral tx.
- **Oral terbinafine** [3]: first-line. A Cochrane review found evidence for superiority of terbinafine over other oral antifungals. Mycological cure rate from meta-analysis ~77%. Fingernails – 250mg OD for 6 weeks; toenails 250mg OD for 12 weeks. RCTs suggest combination with topicals, as above, is superior than oral tx alone.
- **Itraconazole** [3]: second-line, *although it is treatment of choice for yeasts and moulds.* Meta-analysis reported cure rates of 59–75%. Pulsed: fingernails – 200mg BD for 1 week per month for 2 months and for toenails 200mg BD for 1 week per month for 3 months. Continuous therapy: 200mg OD for 6 weeks (fingernails) or 12 weeks (toenails).
- **Other oral antifungals, less efficacious** [3]: fluconazole (150–300mg once weekly ~3–6 months), griseofulvin (500–1000mg/day for 6–9 months fingernails, 12–18 months toenails), posaconazole.
- **Refractory:** laser treatment [4] (poor efficacy in RCTs), PDT [3], nail avulsion [4].

Patients may enquire about **vinegar soaks.** Some authors report vinegar soaks (or soaking and donning a sock) for 15 minutes, prior to the application of topical antifungals, improves clinical response.

Sensitivity and specificity of diagnostic tests for onychomycosis

	Sensitivity	Specificity
KOH	67–93%	38–78%
Fungal culture	31–59%	83–100%
Histopathology with PAS	92%	72%
PCR	95%	100 %

Tinea pedis recurrence rates are very high, approaching 50%.

Preventing and managing recurrence:

- Identifying the organism is key to targeted treatment. Three groups cause onychomycosis – 70% dermatophytes (mostly *T rubrum*), 20% non-dermatophyte moulds (e.g. *Scopulariopsis*), and 10% yeasts (e.g. *Candida*).
- Keep feet cool and dry, avoid occlusive footwear, manage hyperhidrosis.
- Treat affected family members.
- Discard or treat infected footwear.
- Manage nail trauma.
- Use prophylactic antifungals to feet, webs, and nails weekly.
- Consider 'booster' therapy: 4 weeks of terbinafine/itraconazole given 6–9 months after initial tx, in those with severe disease/risk factors/slow to improve.

Urticaria

In general, acute urticaria (<6 weeks) does not require investigation. Chronic spontaneous urticaria (CSU) lasts 6 weeks or more and the management strategy below largely pertains to this.

All Patients

1) **Take a history screening for triggers and systemic symptoms:** drugs (NSAIDs, ACE-I etc.), fever, arthralgias, malaise, physical triggers, and comorbidities.
2) **Bloods:** although guidelines differ, in general patients with CSU not responding to the approved dose of an antihistamine are tested for FBC, ESR/CRP, and TFTs.

Short courses prednisolone ($\leq$0.5mg/kg/d, for 3 days) if necessary for uncontrollable severe symptoms including angioedema of the mouth.

Step 1

- **Single-agent second-generation antihistamine** [4]: cetirizine 10mg/levocetirizine 5mg/fexofenadine 180mg/loratadine 10mg. Usually started at OD/BD for mild–moderate disease and titrated up to × 4 the recommended dose. Ensure patient understands must continue taking medication, even in the absence of symptoms, to prevent relapse. Can be weaned slowly once stable for 2–4 weeks. Some clinicians combine second-generation antihistamines (but little evidence).

Step 2

- **Add montelukast** [4]: 10mg ON. Different studies have shown conflicting evidence for efficacy.
  In some centres, particularly with limited omalizumab access, the following are utilized but poor evidence:
- **Add hydroxyzine** [4]: start at 25mg ON and increase as tolerated. No evidence that adding this increases efficacy, but it is commonly employed.
- **Add H2 antihistamine** [1]: Cochrane review concluded that there was insufficient evidence to recommend, but they are still commonly used. Prescribe famotidine 20mg BD or nizatidine 150–300mg BD.

Handbook of Skin Disease Management, First Edition. Zainab Jiyad and Carsten Flohr.
© 2023 John Wiley & Sons Ltd. Published 2023 by John Wiley & Sons Ltd.
Companion website: www.wiley.com/go/jiyad/handbookofskindiseasemanagement

Refractory

- **Omalizumab** [1]: *treatment of choice* for antihistamine refractory disease. <u>Use 300mg every 4 weeks from 12 years.</u>
- **Ciclosporin** [1]: rapid onset, alternative if omalizumab not effective or evidence of autoimmune urticaria (positive basophil activation assays). Meta-analysis concluded that the overall response rate with low to moderate doses at 4, 8, and 12 weeks was 54%, 66%, and 73%, respectively.
- **Limited evidence:** tacrolimus, MMF, dapsone, sulfasalazine.

Urticarial vasculitis

Complement levels should be checked, though most cases of urticarial vasculitis (UV) are normocomplementaemic. Hypocomplementaemia does not necessarily indicate hypocomplementaemic urticarial vasculitis syndrome (HUVS), which is associated with systemic features, anti-C1q antibodies, and renal disease. In the absence of systemic features, low complement urticarial vasculitis is confusingly termed hypocomplementaemic urticarial vasculitis (HUV) – without the syndrome.

All Patients

1) **History screening for systemic features and drug causes:** fever, aches, GI, respiratory symptoms, CNS, and others.
2) **History and examination screening for associated conditions:** SLE, Sjogren's, infection such as hepatitis, malignancy.
3) **Ix:** FBC, complement levels, CRP, ESR, U/Es, LFTs, ANA, ENA, further screening as directed by history.
4) **Skin biopsy +/- immunofluorescence.**

Course of oral steroids can be used for acute flares, usually as weaning regimen.

Step 1

- **Antihistamines** [3]: commonly used, although a SR found in 76% of cases they were ineffective. Trial H1 antihistamines, e.g. fexofenadine 180mg BD.
- **NSAIDs** [3]: same SR of published studies report some improvement in 35% of patients (of 100 in total).

Step 2

- **Dapsone** [3]: *see page 186 for dosing.* SR concluded that benefit was seen in 63% of patients.
- **Colchicine** [3]: *use 500 micrograms start at OD and increase to BD after 1 week, as tolerated, to maximum of 2mg.* Found to be effective in 36% of cases, based on uncontrolled studies.
- **Hydroxychloroquine** [3]: some benefit reported in 39% of cases. Use 200mg OD or BD aiming for 5mg/kg/d to minimise any long-term risk of retinopathy.

Handbook of Skin Disease Management, First Edition. Zainab Jiyad and Carsten Flohr.
© 2023 John Wiley & Sons Ltd. Published 2023 by John Wiley & Sons Ltd.
Companion website: www.wiley.com/go/jiyad/handbookofskindiseasemanagement

Refractory

- **Methotrexate** [3]: pooling case series/reports shows response in 50% of cases (20 total). *Standard dosing, page 181.*
- **Ciclosporin/MMF/azathioprine** [4]: *see Appendix A for dosing.*
- **Omalizumab** [3]: 15 of 16 total cases derived some benefit, with the majority showing complete remission.
- **Others:** IVIG, anakinra, canakinumab, anti-TNF, thalidomide, (cyclophosphamide for severe end organ damage only).

C

Vasculitis (cutaneous small-vessel) (CSVV)

It is important to distinguish between small, small-medium, medium, or large vessel vasculitis (page 210). The investigations below are relevant to any new suspected case of small-vessel vasculitis; however, the treatment recommended generally pertains to chronic vasculitis. Treatment is only required in *symptomatic* patients.

All Patients

1) **Take a history screening for causes and triggers:** infection, medications, connective tissue diseases, RA, and malignancy.
2) **Perform a punch biopsy with IMF (see page 218):** the identification of IgA vasculitis is important, and biopsy should be undertaken in most patients.
3) **Vasculitis blood screen:** FBC, U+Es, LFTs, +/- following - ANA, complement, ANCA, HIV, Hepatitis B+C, cryoglobulins, rheumatoid factor.
4) **Perform a urine dipstick.**
5) **Check blood pressure.**

Step 1

- **Compression stockings** [4]: leg elevation should also be encouraged.
- **Potent TCS** [4]: may improve symptoms, particularly itch.
- **Oral steroids** [3]: if required, a weaning course is started – 30–40mg, tapered over 4–6 weeks. Evidence for efficacy is based on clinical experience and retrospective reviews.

Step 2

- **Colchicine** [4]: RCT of 41 found no significant difference between colchicine vs emollient. Retrospective reviews and case reports have reported success. 500 micrograms start at OD and increase to BD after 1 week, as tolerated, to maximum of 2mg.
- **Dapsone** [4]: based on case reports. Standard dosing (see page 186).
- **Azathioprine** [4]: case reports suggesting improvement. Standard dosing (see page 185).

Refractory

- **Other immunosuppressants, case reports** [4]: methotrexate, ciclosporin, MMF.
- **Others** [4]: hydroxychloroquine, IVIG, rituximab, minocycline.

Handbook of Skin Disease Management, First Edition. Zainab Jiyad and Carsten Flohr.
© 2023 John Wiley & Sons Ltd. Published 2023 by John Wiley & Sons Ltd.
Companion website: www.wiley.com/go/jiyad/handbookofskindiseasemanagement

Vitiligo

Treatment depends on type of vitiligo (segmental vs generalised) and extent of disease.

All Patients

1) **Check TFTs and thyroid antibodies:** a SR has found high prevalence of thyroid disease with vitiligo, and screening is recommended in all patients.
2) **Assess psychosocial impact:** use vitiligo-specific QoL scales. Refer moderate/severe for psychological therapies, e.g. CBT.
3) **Advise/refer to camouflage services.**
4) **Advise regarding photoprotection:** SPF 50 and 5-star UVA. Vitamin D deficiency is common and levels should be checked.

For unstable vitiligo at any stage, give course of **oral steroids** (oral betamethasone 0.1mg/kg twice weekly on 2 consecutive days for 3 months followed by tapering of the dose by 1mg/month for a further 3 months, ideally in combination with NBUVB). Use alternative steroid if betamethasone if not available (see page 221 for steroid conversion).

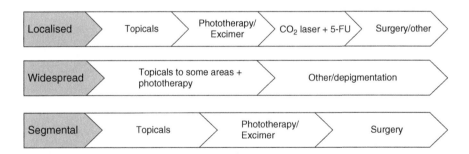

Clinical Pearl

There is growing evidence to suggest that combination treatments achieve better results – e.g. phototherapy and topicals. Consider combining treatments, where appropriate.

Handbook of Skin Disease Management, First Edition. Zainab Jiyad and Carsten Flohr.
© 2023 John Wiley & Sons Ltd. Published 2023 by John Wiley & Sons Ltd.
Companion website: www.wiley.com/go/jiyad/handbookofskindiseasemanagement

Topicals

- **Potent/superpotent TCS** [4]: use OD for 12 weeks. If some improvement, continue with gradual wean/short breaks. *Topical of choice.* Can be used on alternate weeks on thinner skin, +/- tacrolimus on other weeks.
- **Topical tacrolimus** [4]: use BD; particularly beneficial in facial vitiligo.
- **Calcipotriol** [4]: 1 RCT found that topical calcipotriol enhanced phototherapy, whilst another found no improvement. No clear role at present due to lack of evidence.

Phototherapy

- **NBUVB** [1]: *first-line.* Topical tacrolimus or TCS may improve success of repigmentation. A meta-analysis found that almost three-fourths of included patients achieved at least 25% improvement at 6 months.
- **PUVA** [1]: largely superseded by NBUVB but can be used if NBUVB has failed.
- **Excimer lamps/laser** [3]: equally efficacious and similarly efficacious to NBUVB. Best for localised disease.

Surgery

Surgical options should be reserved for segmental vitiligo or stable, non-progressive vitiligo.
- Best evidence for **cellular grafting,** e.g. cultured autologous melanocyte cell suspension.
- **Mini-punch grafting** has been used, though limited evidence.

CO_2 + 5-FU

- **CO_2 laser + topical 5-FU** [4]: may be useful for refractory acral vitiligo. Apply 5-FU once daily for 7 days per month for 5 months with CO_2 laser treatments once a month for 5 months.

Other

- **JAK inhibitors** [3]: most studies have used tofacitinib 5mg OD. A meta-analysis of 45 patients reported >50% improvement in 57.8% of patients. Evidence suggests results are enhanced with concurrent NBUVB.
- **Complementary therapies:** a variety of complementary treatments have been reported, but the evidence is weak and insufficient to recommend these treatments.

Depigmentation

- **Monobenzone/others** [4]: for extensive vitiligo, consider this option after careful discussion with patients.

Vulvodynia

Differentiate from vulval pain secondary to a vulval skin condition. Treatment below pertains to vulval pain of at least 3 months' duration, with no identifiable primary cause.

All Patients

1) Take a **history screening for causes and triggers.**
2) Recommend a **multidisciplinary approach** (physiotherapy, psychotherapy, pain clinic).
3) Recommend **soap substitute and emollients.**
4) **Assess impact on sexual health** (recommend lubricants, if needed).

Clinical Pearl

The cotton-swab test is most widely used. A cotton-tipped applicator is touched against the inner thigh and used as control. Subsequently, it is applied in a circumferential manner to the vestibule. The patient should rate pain on a scale of 1–10 (maximum pain).

Step 1

- **Emollient** [4]: as a soap substitute and regular moisturiser. Recommend avoidance of fragranced products.
- **Topical lidocaine** [4]: although a double-blinded RCT showed no benefit, anecdotally success is reported, and it may be particularly beneficial before intercourse.

Step 2

- **Oral amitriptyline/nortriptyline** [4]: initiate at 5mg and increase in 5mg doses to 20mg, as required. Two RCTs showed no benefit over placebo.
- **SNRIs/SSRIs** [4]: in an open-label trial of 22 women, milnacipran significantly improved pain. Use of duloxetine started at 30mg OD can increase to 60mg, or venlafaxine 75mg OD (if co-existent depression). Less evidence for SSRIs.
- **Topical oestrodiol 0.01% cream** [4]: though evidence is conflicting, in 1 RCT of 39 post-menopausal women, topical oestrodiol was found to significantly reduce symptoms. Apply at bedtime just to the vulvar vestibule.

Handbook of Skin Disease Management, First Edition. Zainab Jiyad and Carsten Flohr.
© 2023 John Wiley & Sons Ltd. Published 2023 by John Wiley & Sons Ltd.
Companion website: www.wiley.com/go/jiyad/handbookofskindiseasemanagement

> **Refractory**
>
> - **Neuropathic pain agents** [4]: <u>gabapentin</u> most studied. Although evidence from case series and uncontrolled studies reported good efficacy, a placebo-controlled RCT of 230 women showed no benefit. <u>Start at 100mg OD, increase to 300mg OD on day 3 and increase as required and where tolerated in 300mg increments to maximum of 3.6g/day.</u> Carbamazepine and pregabalin are alternatives.
> - **Topical capsaicin** [3]: efficacy cannot be determined as observational studies used topical lidocaine as well. Note capsaicin preparations are made with an alcohol base and can worsen vulvodynia.
> - **Botox** [4]: although a randomised trial showed no benefit compared with saline, significant improvement has been reported in uncontrolled studies.

Warts (viral)

Reassurance is essential, and often no treatment is necessary. In general, management is dependent on age (cryotherapy often difficult in children) and site (acral warts require more aggressive treatment). Prognostically, half of warts will resolve in children by 1 year; in adults this can take several years. In immunosuppressed person, warts can be large, widespread, and slow to respond to treatment, and in the absence of known immunosuppression, such warts should prompt a check of immune function.

Step 1

- **Salicylic acid** [1]: variable concentrations available. Higher concentrations used on acral sites (e.g. 50%) and often require compounding in pharmacy. Advise patients to pare wart before using salicylic acid daily with occlusion (duct tape often used). Cochrane review found superiority over placebo, but widely variable success rates. Overall, just over half resolve (vs 37% treated with placebo). Some evidence to suggest combining with cryotherapy for better results.
- **Cryotherapy** [1]: via cryospray or cotton-bud (similar efficacy but cotton-bud allows for greater precision). Best results achieved by repetitive tx every 2–3 weeks. Cochrane review suggests similar efficacy to salicylic acid.

Step 2

- **5% imiquimod** [4]: frequently used for ano-genital warts. Various regimens are used (typically 3 times a week for max 16 weeks), but on sensitive areas (e.g. face, ano-genital) cautious application is recommended: use 2.5% daily until first signs of inflammation develop, then discontinue. When used, the keratin should be removed first with paring or pre-treatment with salicylic acid, to allow penetration.
- **Duct tape** [1]: conflicting evidence for efficacy, but it is relatively easy to trial. Meta-analysis (duct tape vs placebo) found no evidence to recommend.
- **Top 5-FU +/- salicylic acid (e.g. Actikerall® is an unlicensed combination treatment)** [4]: applied once daily for 12 weeks.
- **DPCP** [1]: limited availability. See page 11 for application guide. Cochrane review showed pool RR of 2.12, 95% CI 1.38–3.26. SADBE is alternative if DPCP not available.

Handbook of Skin Disease Management, First Edition. Zainab Jiyad and Carsten Flohr.
© 2023 John Wiley & Sons Ltd. Published 2023 by John Wiley & Sons Ltd.
Companion website: www.wiley.com/go/jiyad/handbookofskindiseasemanagement

> Refractory

- **Surgery** ④: curettage and cautery/shave excisions most commonly used.
- **Trichloroacetic acid** ④: high concentrations (50–80%) applied every 7–10 days have produced clearance in an RCT.
- **Intralesional bleomycin** ④: success rates highly variable and pain is a well-recognised problem. Limited availability.
- **HPV vaccination** ③: in a retrospective review of 30 treated with quadrivalent vaccine, ~two-thirds achieved complete or partial resolution.
- **Other intralesional injections (e.g. MMR vaccine)** ④: some evidence for good response, but limited to very few specialists with experience in performing this.
- **Pulsed-dye laser** ④: in a retrospective review, 86% of 209 achieved complete/near-complete resolution.
- **Photodynamic therapy** ④: conflicting results from RCTs make it unclear to know if it is more effective than placebo.
- **Others:** oral retinoids, cantharidin, podophyllin, intralesional vitamin D, glutaraldehyde, formaldehyde.

Zinc deficiency

The key step in management is determining the cause of zinc deficiency (and treat, where possible), as per the 5 main categories below.

I - Inadequate intake
- Low maternal zinc in breast-fed children
- Eating disorders
- Total parenteral nutrition without zinc supplements

II - Excessive loss
- Fluid losses e.g. diarrhea
- Increased urinary elimination e.g. renal disease
- Blood losses from any cause e.g. parasites

III - Malabsorption
- Acrodermatitis enteropathica
- Coeliac disease
- Inflammatory bowel disease
- Pancreatic dysfunction
- High copper/iron intake

IV - Increased demand
- Pregnancy/breast-feeding
- Preterm infants

V - Other
- Down syndrome
- Congenital thymus defect

Handbook of Skin Disease Management, First Edition. Zainab Jiyad and Carsten Flohr.
© 2023 John Wiley & Sons Ltd. Published 2023 by John Wiley & Sons Ltd.
Companion website: www.wiley.com/go/jiyad/handbookofskindiseasemanagement

Zinc deficiency

Z

Investigations:

- Fasting serum **zinc** level.
- **Alkaline phosphatase** is zinc dependent, and low levels can suggest zinc deficiency, although it can be normal in mild cases.
- Consider checking for **other nutritional deficiencies**, as appropriate, including **copper and iron levels** as these interact with zinc, and high amounts can decrease zinc absorption.
- **Gene testing** if acrodermatitis enteropathica is suspected.

Zinc
replacement

Zinc sulphate 1mg/kg/day (often in divided doses): for acrodermatitis enteropathica this is usually for life, although the dose is guided by serum zinc measurements every 3–6 months. For other causes of zinc deficiency, treat for 6 months usually and correct the underlying cause.

Higher doses 3mg/kg/day are sometimes necessary, particularly for acrodermatitis enteropathica.

Methotrexate

- **Screening tests pre-treatment:** FBC, renal and liver profile, hepatitis B (see page 221 for serology guide) and C, HIV, VZV serology, pregnancy test, quantify alcohol intake. CXR only if hx suggests need for this. TB testing only if hx suggestive.
- **Absolute contraindications:**
- *Immunological:* marrow dysfunction/failure; immunodeficiency states (some, not all); hypersensitivity to MTX.
- *Renal:* severe renal disease or dialysis.
- *Women:* conception, pregnancy, and breastfeeding. Must be off MTX 6 months before conceiving (males too).
- *GI/liver:* severe hepatic dysfunction/cirrhosis; active viral hepatitis; active peptic ulceration.
- *Respiratory:* pulmonary fibrosis or significantly reduced lung function.
- *Other:* active TB; drug interactions.
- **Relative contraindications:** renal impairment (see GFR dose reduction overleaf), liver disease, hepatitis B or C, excessive alcohol intake, gastritis, recent live vaccinations.

Dose
ONCE weekly only dose. Co-prescribe with 5mg folic acid either every day except day of MTX or once weekly (avoiding day of MTX). - Initiate at 5–10mg WEEK 1. - Increase to 15mg WEEK 2. - Maintain at 15mg until review in clinic at WEEK 12. If not improved: increase by 2.5–5mg, otherwise maintain dose. - At doses of 20–22.5mg, consider switching to subcutaneous MTX, if not improving. **(Maximum dose 25mg/week).** - **Paediatric dose is different: 0.4mg/kg/week, max 25mg.**

Monitoring
FBC, U/Es, and LFTs to be checked: - Every 2 weeks until on stable dose: typically pre-treatment, week 2, week 4, and week 12. - Then every 3 months once on stable dose.

Handbook of Skin Disease Management, First Edition. Zainab Jiyad and Carsten Flohr.
© 2023 John Wiley & Sons Ltd. Published 2023 by John Wiley & Sons Ltd.
Companion website: www.wiley.com/go/jiyad/handbookofskindiseasemanagement

Table A.1   Abnormal results and recommended actions.

Total WBC count <3 × 10⁹ cells L⁻¹	Withhold/decrease dose of MTX; consider discussing with haematologist
Neutrophils <10 × 10⁹ cells L⁻¹	Withhold/decrease dose of MTX; consider discussing with haematologist
Platelets <100 × cells L⁻¹	Withhold/decrease dose of MTX; consider discussing with haematologist
MCV >105 fL	Consider withholding/decreasing dose of MTX; check serum B12, folate, and thyroid function tests; consider discussing with haematologist
AST and ALT increased by less than 2 times the normal	Repeat LFTs in 2–4 weeks
AST and ALT greater than 2–3 times the normal	Withhold/decrease dose of MTX; consider other risk factors and consider discussing with gastroenterologist
Nausea and vomiting	Increase folic acid frequency supplementation (6 days a week); consider changing time of day of dose (e.g. night time), antiemetics; switch to subcutaneous MTX
New or increasing dyspnoea or dry cough	Withhold/decrease dose of MTX; repeat chest X-ray and pulmonary function tests and discuss with respiratory team
Severe sore throat, abnormal bruising	Withhold MTX; check FBC immediately; suspect overdose and refer to hospital

Source: Warren RB, Weatherhead SC, Smith CH, et al. British Association of Dermatologists' guidelines for the safe and effective prescribing of methotrexate for skin disease 2016. Br J Dermatol 2016;175(1):23–44.

Table A.2   GFR determines dosage of MTX

>90	Normal dose MTX
20–50	Half-dose MTX
<20	Avoid MTX

A **temporary transaminitis** is often seen with MTX. This does not usually require discontinuation, and rechecking bloods in 2–4 weeks is advised. In a study comparing rheumatological MTX monitoring vs dermatological monitoring, rheumatology monitoring (which is less frequent) meant less discontinuation of MTX and no increase in adverse effects.

Ciclosporin

- **Screening tests pre-treatment:** FBC, renal and liver profile, hepatitis B (see page 221 for serology guide) and C, HIV, VZV, fasting lipids, blood pressure, urine dipstick, weight. CXR and TB test (e.g. TSPOT), usually only if hx suggests need for this.

- **Contraindications/cautions:**
- *Immunological:* marrow dysfunction/failure; immunodeficiency states; previous or current malignancy.
- *Renal impairment.*
- *Women:* conception, pregnancy (can use if benefits outweigh risks), and breastfeeding (avoid).
- *GI/liver:* hepatic dysfunction/cirrhosis.
- *Other:* uncontrolled hypertension; infections; drug interactions.

Dose
Usually given as a BD dose. Capsules come in 25mg, 50mg, and 100mg and different brands. Ensure the same brand is prescribed. Dose ranges from 2 to 5mg/kg/day.   • Initiate at 2.5–5mg/kg/day (depending on disease severity; max. 5mg/kg/day).   • At next review (4–12 weeks), if not improving can increase dose by 0.5–1mg/kg. Alternatively, if markedly improved consider reducing by 0.5mg/kg, otherwise maintain dose if good response.

Monitoring
U/Es and BP (usually FBC and LFTs too) to be checked: • Every 2 weeks for 12 weeks.   • Thereafter, monthly for 1–2 months.   • Then 3 monthly once on stable dose.   Urine dip stick and fasting lipids to be repeated at clinic visits.

Table A.3 Abnormal results and recommended actions.

Rise in creatinine	• Single measurements should always be interpreted with caution, as only sustained changes are clinically important. • If serum creatinine rise >30% above baseline, the test should be repeated within a fortnight. • If the rise is sustained at this level, then the ciclosporin dosage should usually be reduced by at least 1 mg kg^{-1} per day for at least 1 month. • If the value then falls back to less than 30% above baseline, then ciclosporin can be continued at the reduced dosage. • However, should the creatinine level not decrease below the 30% above the patient's baseline value, then ciclosporin should usually be discontinued. Reintroduction of ciclosporin may be considered when renal function returns to within 10% elevation over the patient's baseline value, but if elevation of 30% recurs it should usually be discontinued permanently.
Blood pressure elevation	• Intervene if BP above 140/90 or 130/90 if patient has diabetes/eye disease/renal disease or cerebrovascular disease. • Manage elevation either by reducing the dosage of ciclosporin or by introducing antihypertensive drug therapy.

Source: Berth-Jones J, Exton LS, Ladoyanni E, et al. British Association of Dermatologists' guidelines for the safe and effective prescribing of oral ciclosporin in dermatology 2018. Br J Dermatol 2019;180(6):1312–38.

- **Ciclosporin levels** are not routinely checked, unlike in other specialties. There may be benefit in checking levels in higher doses (4mg/kg +), or where there has been a poor response.
- **The trend of renal function is key** – monitor this and *not* EGFR (which can often be normal despite rising creatinine).

Azathioprine

- **Screening tests pre-treatment:** FBC, TPMT level renal and liver profile, hepatitis B (see page 221 for serology guide) and C, HIV, VZV.
- **Contraindications/cautions:**
- 🚶 *Immunological:* marrow dysfunction/failure; immunodeficiency states; previous or current malignancy.
- 🫘 *Renal impairment.*
- 🚶 *Women:* conception, pregnancy, and breastfeeding (can use if benefits outweigh risks).
- 🫃 *GI/liver:* viral hepatitis.
- 🪝 *Other:* infections; drug interactions, multiple previous skin cancers.

Dose
TPMT level determines dosing, as follows: • TPMT absent: generally considered unsuitable for azathioprine. • TPMT intermediate: 1–1.5mg/kg/day (paediatric dose is 0.5–1.5mg/kg/day). • TPMT normal: 2–3mg/kg/day (paediatric dose is 1–3mg/kg/day).

Monitoring
FBC, U/Es, and LFTs to be checked: • Weekly for first month. • Monthly thereafter. • Then 3 monthly once on stable dose.

Dapsone

- **Screening tests pre-treatment:** FBC, reticulocyte count, MCV, renal and liver profile, G6PD.
- **Contraindications/cautions:**
- ⚕ *Immunological:* hypersensitivity to dapsone; allergy to sulfonamides; G6PD deficiency.
- 🫘 *Renal impairment.*
- ⚕ *Women:* conception, pregnancy, and breastfeeding (can use if benefits outweigh risks).
- 🥄 *GI/liver:* liver impairment.
- 🗡 *Other:* drug interactions; severe anaemia.

Dose
• Initiate at 50mg OD week 1. • Gradually increase to maximum of 300mg/day as required (dose of 1–2mg/kg).

Monitoring

FBC, reticulocyte count, MCV, LFTs, U&Es:
 	
  • Weekly for 1 month.
  • Then every 2 weeks until week 12.
  • Then every 3 months.
 	
Methemoglobin level as clinically indicated (headache, dizziness, etc.).

Table A.4   Abnormal results and recommended actions for dapsone.

>Two-fold rise in aspartate transaminase (AST), alanine transaminase (ALT) (from upper limit of reference range)	Repeat check after 2 weeks. Check for other causes of deranged LFTs, e.g. alcohol excess. If persistently elevated or >four-fold rise, stop dapsone and review.
White cell count <3.5 × 10*9/L **Neutrophils <2 × 10*9/L** **Haemoglobin fall of >20g/L from baseline** **Reticulocyte count increases by >6%** **Platelets <150 × 19*9/L**	Stop dapsone, review and discuss with haematology.
MCV >105 fl	Check B12, folate, and TFTs and start supplementation if low.
▌Methaemoglobin >20%	Stop dapsone and urgent review.
▌Methaemoglobin >30%	Stop dapsone, urgent review, and consider treatment in A&E with methylene blue.

- **Dapsone hypersensitivity syndrome** occurs in 1 in 100, 3–6 weeks after starting dapsone. It presents with fever, rash, and pruritus.
- **Methaemoglobinaemia** is associated with cyanosis, headaches, dyspnoea.
- A degree of **haemolysis** occurs in most patients, but fall in Hb >20g/L should be reviewed.

Mycophenolate Mofetil (MMF)

- **Screening tests pre-treatment:** FBC, renal and liver profile, hepatitis B (see page 221 for serology guide) and C, HIV, VZV, CXR. TB testing if high risk.
- **Contraindications/cautions:**
- 🧍 *Immunological:* active infection or high risk for infection.
- 🧍 *Women:* conception, pregnancy, and breastfeeding.
- 🌢 *GI/liver:* active serious GI disease (risk of haemorrhage, ulceration, and perforation).
- 🗡 *Other:* drug interactions.

Dose
• Start at 500mg BD. • Review at 4 weeks, if no improvement or poor progress, increase in 500mg increments to maximum of 1.5g BD.

Monitoring
FBC (+/- LFTs and U/Es at intervals) to be checked: • Weekly for first month. • Then twice a month for 2 months. • Then monthly for the first year.

Table A.5 Abnormal results and recommended actions for MMF.

Total WBC count $<3 \times 10^9$ cells L^{-1}	Withhold/decrease. Consider discussing with haematologist.
Neutrophils $<10 \times 10^9$ cells L^{-1}	Withhold/decrease. Consider discussing with haematologist.
Platelets $<100 \times$ cells L^{-1}	Withhold/decrease. Consider discussing with haematologist.
MCV >105 fL	Consider withholding/decreasing. Check serum B12, folate, and thyroid function tests; consider discussing with haematologist.
AST and ALT increased by less than 2 times the normal	Repeat LFTs in 2–4 weeks.
AST and ALT greater than 2–3 times the normal	Withhold/decrease dose; consider other risk factors and consider discussing with gastroenterologist.
Oral ulceration, severe sore throat, or abnormal bruising	Withhold dose, review, and check FBC immediately.
Gastrointestinal intolerance	Split total daily dose into multiple daily doses, e.g. 1g BD to 500mg QDS.

Isotretinoin

- **Screening tests pre-treatment:** FBC, renal and liver profile, lipid profile, pregnancy test.
- **Contraindications/cautions:**
- *Immunological:* hypervitaminosis A.
- *Women:* pregnancy (should not become pregnant for 1 month after discontinuation) and breastfeeding.
- *Renal impairment.*
- *Dry eye syndrome.*
- *Liver:* liver disease, hyperlipidaemia, alcohol excess.
- *Other:* mental health issues, diabetes, hypersensitivity, inflammatory bowel disease, peanut/soya allergy (although drug information leaflet advises avoiding in those with allergies, there are many cases of use in those with allergies with no side effects reported).

Dose
<ul><li>Work out maximum cumulative dose (120–150mg/kg) for course, to be given typically over one year.</li><li>Initiate at 20mg (or 0.5mg/kg) and increase up as tolerated. This is variable, some increase after 2 weeks, others after 6–8 weeks, and some remain on low dose.</li><li>Give maximum of 1mg/kg/day.</li></ul>

Monitoring
<ul><li>Multiple studies and meta-analysis now confirm that if baseline bloods and peak dose bloods (at 8 weeks) are normal, no further testing is required.</li><li>If 8-week bloods are abnormal, periodic testing is required.</li><li>If female patients have opted into the Pregnancy Prevention Plan, monthly pregnancy tests are required.</li></ul>

Table A.6   Management of complications.

Acne flare	If severe nodulocystic acne/fulminans, initiate reducing course of prednisolone concurrently (typically 20–30 mg starting dose). Low dose may help reduce significant flares.
Raised triglycerides	Minor elevation – monitor and ensure fasting lipids are tested. Moderate elevation (5–8mg/dL) – reduce dose. Severe rise (>8mg/dL) – consider discontinuing and discussing with metabolic specialist.
AST and ALT increased by less than 3 times the normal	Repeat LFTs.
AST and ALT greater than 3 times the normal	Withhold/decrease dose; consider other risk factors and consider discussing with gastroenterologists.
Pregnancy	Stop isotretinoin and refer to obstetrics/gynaecology urgently.
Dry lips/eyes/epistaxis	Lip moisturiser, eye drops, artificial tears. For epistaxis – saline nasal spray and moisturising ointment to nostrils.

Acitretin

- **Screening tests pre-treatment:** FBC, renal and liver profile, lipid profile, pregnancy test.
- **Contraindications/cautions:**
- *Immunological:* hypervitaminosis A.
- *Women:* avoid in women of childbearing age – due to long half-life, pregnancy must be avoided for 3 years after completing acitretin.
- *Renal impairment.*
- *Dry eye syndrome.*
- *Liver:* liver disease, hyperlipidaemia, alcohol excess.
- *Other:* diabetes, hypersensitivity.

Dose

- Generally start at 25–30mg OD, but lower doses are used in many conditions, e.g. rosacea.
- Increase in increments if poor response.
- Maximum of 1mg/kg/day, or 75mg.

Monitoring

- Check FBC, LFTs every 2–4 weeks for first 2 months, then every 3 months.
- Check lipid profile 4 weeks after starting and then every 3 months.

Table A.7 Management of complications of acitretin.

Raised triglycerides	Minor elevation – monitor and ensure fasting lipids are tested. Moderate elevation (5–8mg/dL) – reduce dose. Severe rise (>8mg/dL) – consider discontinuing and discussing with metabolic specialist.
AST and ALT increased by less than 3 times the normal	Repeat LFTs.
AST and ALT greater than 3 times the normal	Withhold/decrease dose; consider other risk factors and consider discussing with gastroenterologists.
Pregnancy	Stop acitretin and refer to obstetrics/gynaecology urgently.
Dry lips/eyes/epistaxis	Lip moisturiser, eye drops, artificial tears. For epistaxis – saline nasal spray and moisturising ointment to nostrils.

Alitretinoin

- **Screening tests pre-treatment:** FBC, renal and liver profile, lipid profile, pregnancy test.
- **Contraindications/cautions:**
- *Immunological:* hypervitaminosis A.
- *Women:* pregnancy and lactation (should not become pregnant for 1 month after discontinuation).
- *Renal impairment.*
- *Dry eye syndrome.*
- *Liver:* liver disease, hyperlipidaemia, alcohol excess.
- *Other:* diabetes, hypersensitivity, mental health issues, peanut or soya allergy as per isotretinoin.

Dose
• Start at 30mg OD, unless diabetes/hyperlipidaemia in which case start at 10mg. • In UK, clinical response to be assessed at 12 weeks to continue.

Monitoring
• Check FBC, U/Es, LFTs, and lipid profile every 3 months.

See page 191 for management of complications.

Spironolactone

- **Screening tests pre-treatment:** FBC, renal and liver profile, pregnancy test.
- **Contraindications/cautions:**
- *Immunological:* Addison's disease, acute porphyrias.
- *Women:* pregnancy and lactation.
- *Renal impairment, polycystic kidney disease, hyperkalaemia.*
- *Other:* elderly, breast cancer.

Dose
<ul><li>Start at 25–50mg OD (usually 50mg).</li><li>Increase gradually up to doses of 200mg OD (these higher doses can be given in 2 divided doses), as tolerated.</li></ul>

Monitoring
<ul><li>If no comorbidities and <45 years, monitoring is not required as risk of hyperkalaemia very low.</li><li>If criteria above not fulfilled, check FBC, U/Es (renal profile), LFTs at baseline and at intervals.</li></ul>

Biologics

Table B.1 Biologics initiation: screening and investigations.

	Screening	Notes
History		
	TB and risk factors Hepatitis B and C HIV	Active or latent TB should be discussed with TB specialist before initiating. If tx required for latent TB, aim to complete 2 months of tx before starting biologic.
	Malignancy	Weigh up risk–benefit and discuss with cancer specialist.
	Demyelinating disease and other neurological	Avoid anti-TNF.
	Heart failure	Avoid anti-TNF in moderate/severe heart failure (NYHA II–IV).
	Smoking	
	Vaccinations and up-to-date with screening	Do not give live vaccines to people on biologic therapy or to infants (up to 6 months of age) whose mothers have received biologic therapy beyond 16 weeks' gestation. Stop biologic therapy for 6–12 months before giving live vaccines.
	Pregnancy	Consider using certolizumab pegol as a first-line choice for psoriasis when starting biologic therapy in women planning conception. Consider stopping biologic therapy in the second/third trimester.
Investigations		
	Height, weight, BP	
	Psoriasis Epidemiology Screening Tool (PEST score, for PsA)	
	CXR and TB testing	
	FBC, U/Es, LFTs, Hep B/C, HIV, ANA, fasting lipids +/- VZV	Test for Hepatitis B (surface antigen and core antibody), Hepatitis C (IgG); some departments only test high-risk groups.
	Pregnancy test	

Handbook of Skin Disease Management, First Edition. Zainab Jiyad and Carsten Flohr.
© 2023 John Wiley & Sons Ltd. Published 2023 by John Wiley & Sons Ltd.
Companion website: www.wiley.com/go/jiyad/handbookofskindiseasemanagement

Table B.2   Biologics: dosing and cautions

BIOLOGIC	DOSE	% ACHIEVING PASI-90 AT 3–4 MONTHS	PSORIATIC ARTHRITIS	PARTICULAR CAUTIONS
Anti-TNF				
Adalimumab	Initial dose of 80mg SC, followed by 40mg SC given every other week starting 1 week after the initial dose.	41%	✓	Moderate/severe heart failure, multiple sclerosis, or other neuro conditions
Certolizumab pegol	400mg (given as 2 SC injections of 200mg each) at weeks 0, 2, and 4. Maintenance dosing of 200mg every 2 weeks.	41–48%	✓	Moderate/severe heart failure, multiple sclerosis, or other neuro conditions
Etanercept	50mg administered once weekly; alternatively, 50mg given twice weekly may be used for up to 12 weeks followed, if necessary, by a dose of 50mg once weekly.	23%	✓	Moderate/severe heart failure, multiple sclerosis, or other neuro conditions
Infliximab	5mg/kg given as an intravenous infusion followed by additional 5mg/kg infusion doses at 2 and 6 weeks after the first infusion, then every 8 weeks thereafter.	53%	✓	Moderate/severe heart failure, multiple sclerosis
IL12/23				
Ustekinumab	45mg (90mg if >100kg) SC, followed by a 45mg (90mg) dose 4 weeks later, and then every 12 weeks thereafter	46%	Only when anti-TNF has failed	–

(*Continued*)

Table B.2 (Continued)

BIOLOGIC	DOSE	% ACHIEVING PASI-90 AT 3–4 MONTHS	PSORIATIC ARTHRITIS	PARTICULAR CAUTIONS
IL17				
Brodalumab	210mg administered by subcutaneous injection at weeks 0, 1, and 2 followed by 210mg every 2 weeks. Consideration should be given to discontinuing treatment in patients who have shown no response after 12–16 weeks of treatment. Some patients with initial partial response may subsequently improve with continued treatment beyond 16 weeks.	73%	✗ Not licensed	Inflammatory bowel disease, recurrent candidal infection
Ixekizumab	Initial dose of 160mg SC (2 80-mg injections) at week 0, followed by 80mg (1 injection) at weeks 2, 4, 6, 8, 10, and 12, then maintenance dosing of 80mg (1 injection) every 4 weeks	72%	✓	Inflammatory bowel disease, recurrent candidal infection
Secukinumab	300mg of secukinumab SC with initial dosing at weeks 0, 1, 2, and 3, followed by monthly maintenance dosing starting at week 4. Each 300mg dose is given as 2 SC injections of 150mg.	60%	✓	Inflammatory bowel disease, recurrent candidal infection
IL23				
Guselkumab	100mg SC at weeks 0 and 4, followed by maintenance dose every 8 weeks.	68%	✗	–

Table B.2 (Continued)

BIOLOGIC	DOSE	% ACHIEVING PASI-90 AT 3–4 MONTHS	PSORIATIC ARTHRITIS	PARTICULAR CAUTIONS
Risankizumab	150mg (two 75-mg injections) SC at weeks 0, 4, and every 12 weeks thereafter	74%	✕	–
Tildrakizumab	100mg SC at weeks 0 and 4 and every 12 weeks thereafter. In patients with certain characteristics (e.g. high disease burden, body weight ≥90kg), 200mg may provide greater efficacy.	39%	✕	–
IL4/13				
Dupilumab	600mg (two 300-mg injections at different sites) initial dose followed by 300mg every 2 weeks SC.	NA	NA	Conjunctivitis is common, consider risk of helminth infection
Tralokinumab	initially 600mg SC day 1 followed by 300mg every 2 weeks. At prescriber's discretion, every fourth week dosing may be considered for patients who achieve clear or almost clear skin after 16 weeks of treatment.	NA	NA	Upper respiratory tract infections; conjunctitivitis
JAK inhibitors				
Abrocitinib	100 mg or 200 mg daily doses, with the lower dose recommended for adolescents as a starting dose.	NA	NA	Abdominal pain, acne, dizziness, nausea, increase in LDL cholesterol, lymphopenia, herpes virus infections

(Continued)

Table B.2 (Continued)

BIOLOGIC	DOSE	% ACHIEVING PASI-90 AT 3–4 MONTHS	PSORIATIC ARTHRITIS	PARTICULAR CAUTIONS
Baracitinib	4mg per day, reduction to 2mg per day possible, depending on treatment response.	NA	NA	Upper respiratory tract infections, increase in LDL cholesterol, thrombocytosis, nausea and abdominal pain, herpes virus infections, acne
Upadacitinib	Adults: 15 or 30mg per day; age ≥65: 15mg per day; age 12–17 (≥30kg): 15mg per day.	NA	NA	Upper respiratory tract infections, acne, headache, anaemia and neutropenia, CK elevation, increase in LDL cholesterol, nausea and abdominal pain, herpes virus infections

Table B.3 Suggested dose-escalation/interval-reduction strategy (local restrictions may apply).

Biological agent	Suggested dose-escalation/interval-reduction strategy
Adalimumab 40mg every other week	Adalimumab 40mg weekly
Certolizumab pegol 200mg every 2 weeks	Certolizumab pegol 400mg every 2 weeks
Etanercept 50mg once weekly	Etanercept 50mg twice weekly
Infliximab 5 mg kg^{-1} every 8 weeks	Infliximab 5 mg kg^{-1} every 6 weeks*
Ixekizumab 80mg every 4 weeks	Ixekizumab 80mg every 2 weeks*
Tildrakizumab 100mg every 12 weeks	Tildrakizumab 200mg every 12 weeks (high disease burden or ≥90kg)
Ustekinumab 45mg every 12 weeks (≤100kg)	Ustekinumab 90mg every 8 or 12 weeks (≤100kg)*
Ustekinumab 90mg every 12 weeks (>100kg)	Ustekinumab 90mg every 8 weeks (>100kg)*

* Off-license use.

Source: Smith CH, Yiu ZZN, Bale T, et al. British Association of Dermatologists guidelines for biologic therapy for psoriasis 2020: a rapid update. Br J Dermatol. 2020;183(4):628–637. doi:10.1111/bjd.19039.

ESSENTIAL LISTS. Many adapted from: Bolognia JL et al., 2012 / With permission of Elsevier.

Causes of annular/arcuate/figurate rash

Childhood/genetic
- Annular erythema of infancy
- Erythrokeratoderma variabilis
- Ichthyosis linearis circumflexa
- Annular lichenoid dermatosis of youth
- EB simplex (Dowling-Meara)
- Annular epidermolytic ichthyosis
- Acute haemorrhagic oedema of infancy
- Elastosis perforans serpiginosa

Papulosquamous
- Annular psoriasis
- Annular seborrheic dermatitis
- Pityriasis rosea
- Pityriasis rotunda
- Pityriasis rubra pilaris
- Annular lichen planus

Infective
- Leprosy
- Syphilis
- Tinea
- Larva migrans
- Larva currens
- Leishmaniasis

Granulomatous
- Sarcoidosis
- Annular elastolytic giant cell granulomatosis
- Granuloma annulare

Handbook of Skin Disease Management, First Edition. Zainab Jiyad and Carsten Flohr.
© 2023 John Wiley & Sons Ltd. Published 2023 by John Wiley & Sons Ltd.
Companion website: www.wiley.com/go/jiyad/handbookofskindiseasemanagement

Figurate erythemas
- Erythema annulare centrifugum
- Erythema marginatum
- Erythema gyratum repens
- Erythema chronicum migrans

Derm-rheum
- Annular erythema of Sjogren's
- Lupus erythematosus
- Jessner's lymphocytic infiltrate

Other
- Well's syndrome
- Erythema multiforme
- Annular capillaritis
- Sneddon-Wilkinson
- Urticarial vasculitis
- Annular urticaria
- Linear IgA disease
- Mycosis fungoides

Causes of telengiectasia

Primary
- Spider naevi
- Hereditary benign telangiectasia
- Generalised essential telengiectasia
- Costal fringe
- Angioma serpiginosum
- Unilateral naevoid telangiectasia
- Cutaneous collagenous vasculopathy

Secondary
- Photodamage
- Post-radiotherapy
- Venous hypertension
- Drugs: oestrogens, steroids, others

Systemic disease
- Carcinoid syndrome
- Telengiectasia macularis eruptive perstans (TMEP)
- Connective tissue diseases
- Mycosis fungoides
- GVHD
- B-cell lymphoma
- Angiolupoid sarcoidosis

Congenital/genodermatoses
- Cutis marmorata
- Hereditory haemorrhagic telangiectasia
- Ataxia-telengiectasia
- Xeroderma pigmentosum
- Rombo syndrome
- Bloom syndrome
- Rothmund-Thompson
- Dyskeratosis congenita
- Poikiloderma with neutropenia
- Goltz syndrome

Causes of sporotrichoid spread

- TB
- Atypical mycobacteria
- Sporotrichosis
- Cat scratch disease
- Tularaemia
- Glanders
- Dimorphic fungi
- Opportunistic fungi
- Anthrax
- Nocardiasis
- Leishmaniasis

Angiokeratoma types

- Angiokeratoma of Fordyce
- Angiokeratoma corporis diffusum
- Angiokeratoma of Mibelli
- Angiokeratoma circumscriptum
- Solitary/multiple

Painful tumours – BENGAL

- Blue rubber bleb naevus
- Eccrine spiroadenoma
- Neuroma, neurolemoma
- Glomus tumour
- Angiolipoma
- Leiomyoma

Causes of multiple lentigines

Localised
- Peutz-Jeghers syndrome
- Bandler syndrome
- Laugier-Hunziker syndrome
- Cantu syndrome
- Cowden syndrome
- Centrofacial lentiginosis
- Inherited patterned lentiginosis
- Cronkhite-Canada syndrome
- Bannayan-Riley-Ruvalcaba
- Xeroderma pigmentosum
- Partial unilateral lentiginosis

Generalised
- LEOPARD syndrome
- Generalised lentiginosis
- Deafness plus lentiginosis
- Carney complex (NAME/LAMB)
- Arterial dissection plus lentiginosis
- Gastrocutaneous syndrome
- Tay syndrome
- Pipkin syndrome

Causes of cold-induced eruptions

- Perniosis
- Chilblain lupus
- Acrocyanosis
- Raynaud's
- Cold panniculitis
- Livedo reticularis
- Cold urticaria
- Cryogobulins
- Cryofibrinogens
- Cold agglutinins

Causes of hypertrichosis

Localised
- Congenital melanocytic naevus
- Becker's naevus
- Plexiform neurofibroma
- Naevoid hypertrichosis
- Smooth muscle hamartoma
- Spinal hypertrichosis
- Anterior/posterior cervical hypertrichosis
- Hypertrichosis of the auricle
- Rubinstein-Taybi syndrome
- Hypertrichosis cubitii
- Cornealia de Lange syndrome
- Repetitive trauma, plaster casting
- Porphyria cutanea tarda
- Following PUVA

Generalised
- Congenital generalised hypertrichosis
- Congenital hypertrichosis languinosa
- Aquired hypertrichosis languinosa
- Prepubertal hypertrichosis
- Congenital adrenal hyperplasia
- Congenital hypothyroidism or maternal drug use
- Drugs: phenytoin, ciclosporin, others
- Hypothyroidism
- HIV
- POEMS syndrome
- Other rare genetic disorders

Causes of scarring alopecias

Lymohocytic
- Lichen planopilaris
- Frontal fibrosing alopecia
- Discoid lupus
- Central centrifugal cicatricial alopecia
- Alopecia mucinosa
- Keratosis follicularis spinulosa decalvans
- GVHD
- Pseudopelade of Brocq

Neutrophilic
- Dissecting cellulitis of the scalp
- Folliculitis decalvans

Mixed
- Acne keloidalis
- Acne necrotica
- Erosive pustular dermatosis of the scalp

Other
- Cicatricial pemphigoid
- Busulphan-induced alopecia
- End-stage traction alopecia

Causes of non-scarring alopecias

- Telogen effluvium
- Androgenetic alopecia
- Alopecia areata
- Trichotillomania
- Psoriasis
- Temporal triangular alopecia
- Lipoedematous alopecia
- Post-operative alopecia

Causes of onycholysis

- Irritants/trauma/UV/water
- Psoriasis
- Infection (HPV, fungal)
- Tetracyclines
- Taxanes
- Hyperthyroidism
- Subungal exostosis
- SCC

Causes of melanonychia

- Racial variation
- Pregnancy
- Trauma
- Drugs: zidovudine, psoralen, chemotherapy
- Nail matrix naevus
- Melanoma
- Laugier-Hunziker
- Addison's disease
- HIV
- Post-inflammatory
- Bowen's disease

Causes of guttate leucoderma

- Idiopathic guttate hypomelanosis
- Pitryriasis versicolor
- Pityriasis lichenoides chronica
- Lichen sclerosus
- Tuberous sclerosus
- Vitiligo ponctué
- Achromic plane warts
- Hypopigmented Darier disease
- Xeroderma pigmentosum
- Clear cell papulosis

Causes of drug-induced acne

- Steroids
- Bromides, iodides
- EGFR inhibitors
- Isoniazid
- Lithium
- Phenytoin
- Progestins
- Ciclosporin
- Azathioprine

Causes of linear dermatoses

- Linear psoriasis
- Linear LP
- Lichen striatus
- Linear lichen sclerosus
- Linear porokeratosis
- Linear Darier disease
- Segmental vitiligo
- Epidermal naevus
- Linear naevoid hypopigmentation
- Pigmentary mosaicism
- HIV
- Incontenentia pigmenti
- Goltz syndrome
- Linear fixed drug eruption
- Linear atrophoderma of Moulin
- Menkes disease
- Corticosteroid injections
- Flagellate erythema
- Pigmentary demarcation lines

Causes of panniculitis

- Erythema nodosum
- Erythema induratum
- Childhood panniculitides:
  - sclerema neonatorum
  - subcutaneous fat necrosis of the newborn
  - post-steroid panniculitis
- Subacute nodular migratory panniculitis
- Injection-related
- Factitial panniculitis
- Lupus panniculitis
- Dermatomyositis-associated panniculitis
- Cold panniculitis
- Morphea
- Pancreatic panniculitis
- Alpha-1 antitrypsin deficiency
- Lipodermatosclerosis
- Panniculitis-like T-cell lymphoma
- Cytophagic haemophagocytic panniculitis
- Idiopathic neutrophilic lobular panniculitis

Photosensitivity dermatoses

Primary
- Polymorphic light eruption
- Juvenile spring eruption
- Chronic actinic dermatitis
- Actinic prurigo
- Solar urticaria
- Actinic folliculitis
- Hydroa vacciniforme

Genetic
- Xeroderma pigmentosum
- Bloom syndrome
- Rothmund-Thompson
- Cockayne syndrome

External
- Drug-induced photosensitivity
- Photocontact dermatitis
- Pseudoporphyria

Metabolic
- Porphyrias

Photoaggravated dermatoses

- Atopic dermatitis
- Bullous pemphigoid
- Carcinoid syndrome
- Cutaneous T cell lymphoma
- Dermatomyositis
- Erythema multiforme
- Darier disease
- Grover's disease
- Lichen planus
- Lupus erythematosus
- Pellagra
- Pemphigus
- Psoriasis
- Rosacea
- Seborrhoeic dermatitis
- Viral infections, e.g. HSV

Causes of café-au-lait macules

- Neurofibromatosis 1 and 2
- Segmental neurofibromatosis
- McCune-Albright
- Legius syndrome
- Noonan syndrome
- Fanconi anaemia
- Bloom syndrome
- Tuberous sclerosis
- PTEN hamartoma-tumour syndrome

C

Vesicular/pustular eruptions in neonates

Infections
- Bacterial (e.g. bullous impetigo)
- Congenital or neonatal candidiasis
- Viruses: HSV, VZV
- Scabies

Transient
- Erythema toxicum neonatorum
- Miliaria
- Neonatal cephalic pustulosis

Other
- Infantile acropustulosis
- Mastocytosis
- Aplasia cutis
- Sucking blister
- Epidermolysis bullosa
- Autoimmune bullous diseases
- Langerhan's histiocytosis
- Congenital erosive and vesicular dermatosis

Vasculopathic disease (micro-occlusive)

Embolic
- Infective endocarditis
- Other septic emboli
- Cholesterol emboli
- Atrial myxoma
- Libman-Sacks endocarditis
- Marantic endocarditis
- Hypereosinophilic syndrome

Coagulopathies
- Purpura fulminans
- Warfarin necrosis
- Antiphospholipid syndrome
- Sneddon syndrome
- Livedoid vasculopathy
- Degos disease
- Protein C / S deficiency
- Factor V leiden

Platelet plugs and cell occlusion
- Heparin-induced thrombocytopenia
- Paroxysmal nocturnal haemoglobinuria
- Thrombocytosis secondary to myeloproliferative disorders
- Thrombotic thrombocytopenic purpura
- Sickle cell disease
- Haemolytic anaemias
- Intravascular lymphoma

Infective
- Vessel-invasive fungi
- Strongyloidiasis
- Ecthyma gangrenosum
- Lucio's phenomenon

Other
- Caciphylaxis
- Hydroxyurea-related
- Brown-recluse spider bite

Cold-related
- Cryoglobulinaemia
- Cryofibrinogenemia
- Cold agglutinins

Vasculitic disease

Small vessel
- Cutaneous small-vessel vasculitis (drugs, infections, malignancies)
- IgA Vasculitis (Henoch-Schonlein purpura)
- Acute haemorrhagic oedema of infancy
- Erythema elevatum diutinum
- Urticarial vasculitis

Small and medium-vessel
- Cryoglobulinaemia
- ANCA +ve vasculitides
- Connective tissue diseases

Medium-vessel
- Polyarteritis nodosa (PAN)

Large-vessel
- Temporal arteritis
- Takayasu's

Blistering/vesicular eruptions

Autoimmune
- Bullous pemphigoid
- Mucous membrane pemphigoid
- Pemphigoid gestationis
- Linear IgA disease
- Epidermolysis bullosa
- Pemphigus
- Bullous lupus
- Bullous vasculitis

Infections
- HSV
- Shingles
- VZV
- Staphylococcal scalded skin syndrome
- Bullous tinea

Drugs
- SJS/TEN

Bland
- Coma blisters
- Bullous diabeticorum
- Oedema blisters
- Friction blisters
- Sucking blister

Photodistributed
- Polymorphic light eruption
- Porphyria
- Pseudoporphyria
- Phototoxic reaction
- Hydroa vacciniforme
- Juvenile spring eruption
- Bullous lupus

Other
- Pompholyx
- Erythema multiforme
- Phytophotodermatitis
- Contact dermatitis
- Sweet's syndrome
- Miliaria

Lymphoedema causes

PRIMARY CAUSES

Syndromic
- Noonan
- Turner
- Costello

Associated with cutaneous/vascular manifestations or disturbed growth
- Proteus
- CLOVE/fibroadipose hyperplasia
- Klippel-Trenaunay/KT-like
- Parkes-Weber syndrome
- WILD syndrome
- Lymphangioma
- Lymphangiomatosis

Congenital onset
- Congenital unisegmental oedema
- Milroy disease
- Lower limb + genital oedema

Other
- GATA2 deficiency
- Lymphoedema-distichiasis syndrome
- Meige and Meige-like
- Late onset multisegmental lymphoedema
- Late onset unilateral leg lymphoedema
- Hennekam syndrome
- Multisegmental lymphatic dysplasia
- Yellow nail syndrome

SECONDARY CAUSES

- Parasitic infections, e.g. filariasis
- Recurrent cellulitis
- Recurrent lymphangitis
- Obesity
- Lymph node dissection (e.g. for breast cancer treatment)
- Malignant obstruction
- Morbihan syndrome (acne/rosacea)
- Granulomatous disease
- Radiation injury
- Podoconiosis

Hurley scoring:

Stage 1: solitary or multiple, isolated abscess formation without scarring or sinus tracts.

Stage 2: recurrent abscesses, single or multiple widely separated lesions, with sinus tract formation.

Stage 3: diffuse or broad involvement, with multiple interconnected sinus tracts and abscesses.

The Hidradenitis Suppurativa Clinical Response (HiSCR)

Defined as at least a 50% reduction in the total number of inflammatory lesions (AN, total count of abscesses and inflammatory nodules) with no increase in abscess count and no increase in draining fistula count relative to baseline.

Fingertip units

Table D.1 Fingertip units.

	Face and neck	Arm and hand	Leg and foot	Trunk front	Back and buttocks
3–12 months	1	1	1.5	1	1.5
1–2 years	1.5	1.5	2	2	3
3–5 years	1.5	2	3	3	3.5
6–10 years	2	2.5	4.5	3.5	5
10 years + (including adults)	2.5	3 for 1 arm 1 for 1 hand	6 for 1 leg 2 for 1 foot	7	7

Handbook of Skin Disease Management, First Edition. Zainab Jiyad and Carsten Flohr.
© 2023 John Wiley & Sons Ltd. Published 2023 by John Wiley & Sons Ltd.
Companion website: www.wiley.com/go/jiyad/handbookofskindiseasemanagement

Table D.2 Dermoscopy methods/checklists.

7-Point Checklist	Menzies Method	3-Point Checklist
Major criteria (2 points each): • Atypical pigment network • Blue-white veil • Atypical vascular pattern	Absence of pattern symmetry AND colour uniformity	1 point each: • Asymmetry • Atypical pigment network • Blue-white structures
Minor criteria: • Irregular streaks • Irregular pigmentation • Irregular dots/ globules • Regression structures	And at least one of the following: • Blue-white veil • Multiple brown dots • Pseudopods • Radial streaming • Scarlike depigmentation • Peripheral black dots/globules • 5–6 colours • Multiple blue/gray dots • Broadened network	
Concerning for melanoma if 3 or more points	Concerning for melanoma if meets major criteria and one of minor criteria	Concerning for melanoma if score of 2 or 3

Hair camouflage

Concealers are temporary and can help considerably with various hair conditions. A variety are available:

• Coloured shampoos
• Coloured mousses and setting lotions
• Creams or wax pencils
• Synthetic fibres – *most commonly used/recommended.*

Available from some pharmacies, but you can direct patients to commonly used brands and websites: Toppik®, Nanogen®, Caboki®, Febron®.

Hair pull test

TEST:

- Grasp 20–60 hairs with your thumb/forefinger.
- Apply constant, gentle pressure and pull from the proximal end to distal end of the hairs.

INTERPRETATION:

- More than 6 hairs pulled away is abnormal and active hair shedding.

Common hairstyles for afro-textured hair

- **Relaxed hair:** an alkaline cream is applied to the hair, causing permanent straightening. Relaxer will need to be reapplied to new hair growth, which should be done every 6–10 weeks.
- **Braids:** hair can be braided in several different ways (box braids, braided twists, knotless braids, etc.). The hair is divided into sections and braided with or without artificial extensions. Cornrows are a type of braid where the hair is braided flat to the scalp in stationary rows.
- **Weaves and extensions:** the native hair is braided into linear cornrows, and pieces of hair that have been wefted together into lines (known as tracks) are sown, glued, or clipped to the native hair.
- **Wigs:** wigs can be worn directly over hair that has been braided into cornrows or twists, or can be worn over a wig cap. Adhesives are sometimes used to secure the wig in place.
- **Dreadlocks:** dreadlocks are rope-like strands, created by twisting hair until it becomes matted in individual threads.

Maintaining afro-textured hair – tips to advise patients

- Two common causes of hair loss in black men/women related to hair care practices are **traction alopecia and acquired trichorrhexis nodosa**. Traction alopecia is caused by sustained or recurring pulling forces on hair follicles, causing hair to be prematurely uprooted. Acquired trichorrhexis nodosa is typified by broken hair shafts caused by extrinsic insults such as heat or chemicals.
- Afro-textured hair needs more moisture, so **a routine for moisturising and conditioning should be developed.**
- Hair should be **washed every 1–2 weeks.**
- More manipulation = more damage. For example, relaxing the hair, dying, and then braiding the hair will significantly increase the risk of both traction alopecia and acquired trichorrhexis nodosa. Some recommend at least a **2-week gap between relaxing and dying hair, and a 2-week gap between relaxing and straightening with heat.**
- **Hair relaxers** should only be applied to new growth and never to hair that has already been straightened.
- Taking **6–12-month breaks from hair relaxers, braids, and thermal straightening** should be considered to give the hair a rest.
- Tight braids, ponytails, and buns increase the risk of traction alopecia. Hair should never be painful, and women should not have to use painkillers after having their hair styled. **Symptoms of pain, stinging, crusting, papules, and/or pustules after hair styling correspond to increased risk of traction alopecia.**
- **Hair adhesives** can cause irritant or contact dermatitis of the scalp.
- **Wigs can rub** on the periphery of the hairline, causing friction and damage to the hair. If wig caps are worn, ones made of satin are less likely to cause frictional damage than ones made of cotton or nylon.
- **Dreadlocks can grow long and heavy**, placing tension on the scalp and increasing the risk of traction alopecia.

Non-scarring alopecia biopsy protocol

Non-scarring protocol:

- 4-mm punch biopsy from affected area.
- 4-mm punch biopsy from control area (usually occiput).
- Send in separate labelled pots.

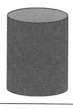
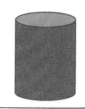

| Involved area | Control area (occiput) |

Scarring alopecia biopsy protocol

Scarring protocol:

- Take x 2 4-mm punch biopsies from the edge of the affected area. Use trichoscopy to identify characteristic features to guide biopsy site. Avoid the 'burnt-out' scarred area.
- Bisect one of the above biopsies in half – send half for immunofluorescence and send the other half with the complete other 4-mm punch biopsy, specifying the need for horizontal and vertical sectioning.

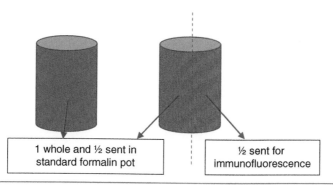

| 1 whole and ½ sent in standard formalin pot | ½ sent for immunofluorescence |

How to biopsy vasculitis

- To ensure that histology is representative, early samples (ideally <24-hrs old) should be taken.
- **Lesional (involved)** skin immunofluorescence is sent.
- Where medium-vessel disease is suspected, a deep biopsy to include subcutis must be taken. This is best done with an incisional biopsy.

How to biopsy a blistering eruption

- Key is to preserve the blister and not deroof.
- If a blister is very small, a punch biopsy around the blister can be taken. Otherwise, the majority of the time an incisional biopsy is done from the edge of the blister.
- **Perilesional (uninvolved)** skin should be sent for immunofluorescence.

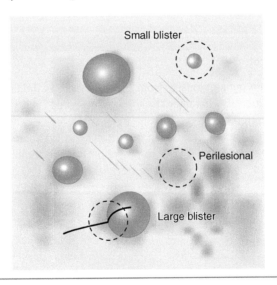

How to biopsy connective tissue disorders

- Take a sample from a representative active area, ideally one that has most recently developed. Where panniculitis is suspected, a deep biopsy to the subcutis is necessary.
- **Lesional (affected skin)** immunofluorescence is sent.

Table D.3 Topical steroid preparations by potency.

Drug	Additions
Mild	
Hydrocortisone (0.1–2.5%)	Canesten HC® (+ clotrimazole)
	Daktacort® (+ miconazole)
	Econacort® (+ econazole)
	Fucidin H® (+ fusidic acid)
	Timodine® (+ dimeticone, nystatin, and benzalkonium chloride)
	Terra-Cotril® (+ oxytetracycline)
Fluocinolone acetonide (Synalar 1 in 10®)	
Moderate	
Betamethasone valerate RD (Betnovate-RD®)	Alphaderm® (+ 10% urea)
Clobetasone butyrate 0.05% (Eumovate®, Clobavate®)	Trimovate® (+ nystatin and oxytetracycline)
Fluticasone propionate (USA)	
Fludroxycortide (Haelan®)	
Alclometasone dipropionate (Modrasone®)	
Fluocinolone acetonide 0.001% (Synalar 1 in 4®)	
Fluocortolone (Ultralanum Plain®)	
Triamcinolone acetonide (USA)	
Potent	
Betamethasone valerate 0.1% (Betnovate®, Betacap® ⬤, Bettamouse®, Betesil plaster®)	Betnovate-N® (+ neomycin)
	Betnovate-® (+ clioquinol)
	Fucibet® (+ fusidic acid)
Beclometasone dipropionate 0.025% (Diprosone®)	Lotriderm® (+ clotrimazole)
	Diprosalic® (+ salicylic acid 3%) + scalp prep available ⬤
	Dovobet®/Enstilar® (+ calcipotriol)
Mometasone furoate 0.1% (Elocon®, Elocon scalp application® ⬤)	
Fluticasone propionate 0.05% (Cutivate®)	
Hydrocortisone butyrate 0.1% (Locoid®, Locoid Crelo® ⬤)	
Fluocinonide 0.05% (Metosyn®)	
Diflucortolone valerate 0.1% (Nerisone®)	
Fluocinolone acetonide 0.025% (Synalar®)	Synalar C® (+ clioquinol)
	Synalar N® (+ neomycin)

(Continued)

Table D.3 (Continued)

Drug	Additions
Super potent	
Clobetasol propionate 0.05% (Dermovate®, Clarelux®, Etrivex shampoo® 🦱)	Dermovate-NN® (+ neomycin and nystatin)
Diflucortolone valerate 0.3% (Nerisone Forte®)	

🦱 = scalp preparations.

Table D.4 Topical antifungals.

Category	Drug	Forms
Azoles	Clotrimazole	Pessary, cream, liquid, spray) E.g. Canesten®
	Ketoconazole	Cream, shampoo E.g. Nizoral®
	Econazole	Pessary, cream E.g. Pevaryl®
	Miconazole	Oromucosal gel, cream, spray, powder E.g. Darkarin®
Allylamines	Terbinafine	Cream E.g. Lamisil®
	Naftifin	Cream and gel Not available in UK
Nail agents	Efinaconazole	E.g. Jublia®
	Amorolfine	E.g. Loceryl®
	Ciclopirox	
	Tavaborole	
	Tioconazole	
Others	Tolnaftate	
	Butenafine	
	Nystatin	

Table D.5 Systemic corticosteroid dose equivalents.

Cortisone	25mg
Hydrocortisone	20mg
Prednisone/prednisolone	5mg
Methylprednisolone	4mg
Triamcinolone	4mg
Betamethasone	0.6–0.75mg
Dexamethasone	0.75mg

Table D.6 Hepatitis B serology.

	Hepatitis B surface antigen (HbsAg)	Hepatitis B surface antibody (anti-HBs)	Hepatitis B Core antibody (anti-HBc)
Susceptible	−ve	−ve	−ve
Vaccinated	−ve	+ve	−ve
Past infection	−ve	+ve	+ve
Acute infection	+ve	−ve	IgM +ve
Chronic infection	+ve	−ve	IgG +ve

Index

Note: Individual drugs have <u>not</u> been indexed for each condition, as readers are advised to seek the specific condition, and then follow the treatment 'steps'. The appendices have been indexed.

Handbook of Skin Disease Management, First Edition. Zainab Jiyad and Carsten Flohr.
© 2023 John Wiley & Sons Ltd. Published 2023 by John Wiley & Sons Ltd.
Companion website: www.wiley.com/go/jiyad/handbookofskindiseasemanagement

Printed and bound by CPI Group (UK) Ltd, Croydon, CR0 4YY

26/02/2024

14459639-0001